THE BIO-PLAN FOR LIFELONG WEIGHT CONTROL

Naola VanOrden, Ph.D
and S. Paul Steed, Ph.D

THE BIO-PLAN FOR LIFELONG WEIGHT CONTROL

*Naola VanOrden, Ph.D
and S. Paul Steed, Ph.D*

THE DIAL PRESS • NEW YORK

Published by
The Dial Press
1 Dag Hammarskjold Plaza
New York, New York 10017

Copyright © 1983 Naola VanOrden and S. Paul Steed
All rights reserved.
Manufactured in the United States of America
First printing

Design by Paul Chevannes

Illustrations by Lindsay Barrett for Pencils Portfolio

Library of Congress Cataloging in Publication Data

VanOrden, Naola.
  The bio-plan for lifelong weight control.

  Includes index.
  1. Reducing diets. 2. Nutrition. 3. Reducing
exercises. 4. Metabolism. I. Steed, S. Paul.
II. Title.
RM222.2.V34   613.2′5   82-1554
ISBN 0-385-27665-6   AACR2

CONTENTS

PART III. SPECIAL ENERGY NEEDS

APPENDIX A. SOURCE NOTES

APPENDIX B. CHARTS AND TABLES

APPENDIX C. BLANK RECORD FORMS

List of Figures

Introduction

Have you ever wondered where all the miracle diets come from? Why do most of them enjoy intense bursts of popularity, and then quickly fade from the scene? Why do none of them seem to provide anything more than a short-term weight loss? Has it seemed to you that all the diets appear to have some common origin? Have you ever suspected that there is a pool of dietary truths into which diet-book authors dip to fashion their own "unique, new, special . . ." diet?

If you have, you are right. Diet-book authors are aware of the chemical and biological laws that govern the functioning of the human body. It is these truths that are packaged in various combinations of emphasis to provide the variety of diets. In most diet books the one or two truths that underlie that particular diet are alluded to and sometimes even explained. But for you to develop a weight-control program that is comfortably realistic and effective, you need more than an occasional glimpse into the pool of dietary truths. You must understand the major "truths" about your body, and how they relate to each other. Once you have that understanding, you will be able to establish a new way of living that will be based on knowledge rather than blind faith and desperate hope. Because you understand why you are making those changes in your life, and because those changes are so carefully tailored to *your* needs, the changes will have great staying power and maximum effect.

We have divided our book into three sections. In the first we describe the chemical and biological laws that govern your body. In the second we provide the instructions, reference tables, and recording forms that you can use to fashion your own weight-control program. In the third section we discuss weight control during adolescence and during pregnancy—periods of life when the need for energy and nutrients is much greater than normal.

Learn the principles. Devise your program. Live your program. You will find that your weight will drop, your shape will change, and your health will improve. Your self-confidence will also increase, and you will enjoy greater peace of mind.

PART I.

Body Chemistry

CHAPTER 1

What Makes People Fat?

We are all aware of some people who never count calories, who seem to eat whatever they like, and yet never gain weight. Then there are other people who must diet continually just to hold their own. Why the difference? Why are some people fat and others thin?

The weight of an animal or person depends upon a finely tuned balance between food intake and food utilization in the body. Adult animals, when not confined to a pen or a cage or a house, keep a remarkably constant body weight most of their lives. Research has shown that adult humans also tend to maintain a fairly stable body weight, whether it is high, normal, or low. In some research studies, when normal-weight volunteers ate very large amounts of food, they were able to gain weight; but they lost the weight shortly after the experiment was discontinued. Likewise, when overweight persons dieted, they lost weight, but regained the weight quickly after discontinuing the diet. These results imply that no crash diet will bring about a permanent weight loss for an overweight person. Only a permanent, comfortable change in life-style can accomplish that.

What, then, determines whether a person will have a high, normal, or low stable body weight? The answer seems to lie in the level of a person's activity

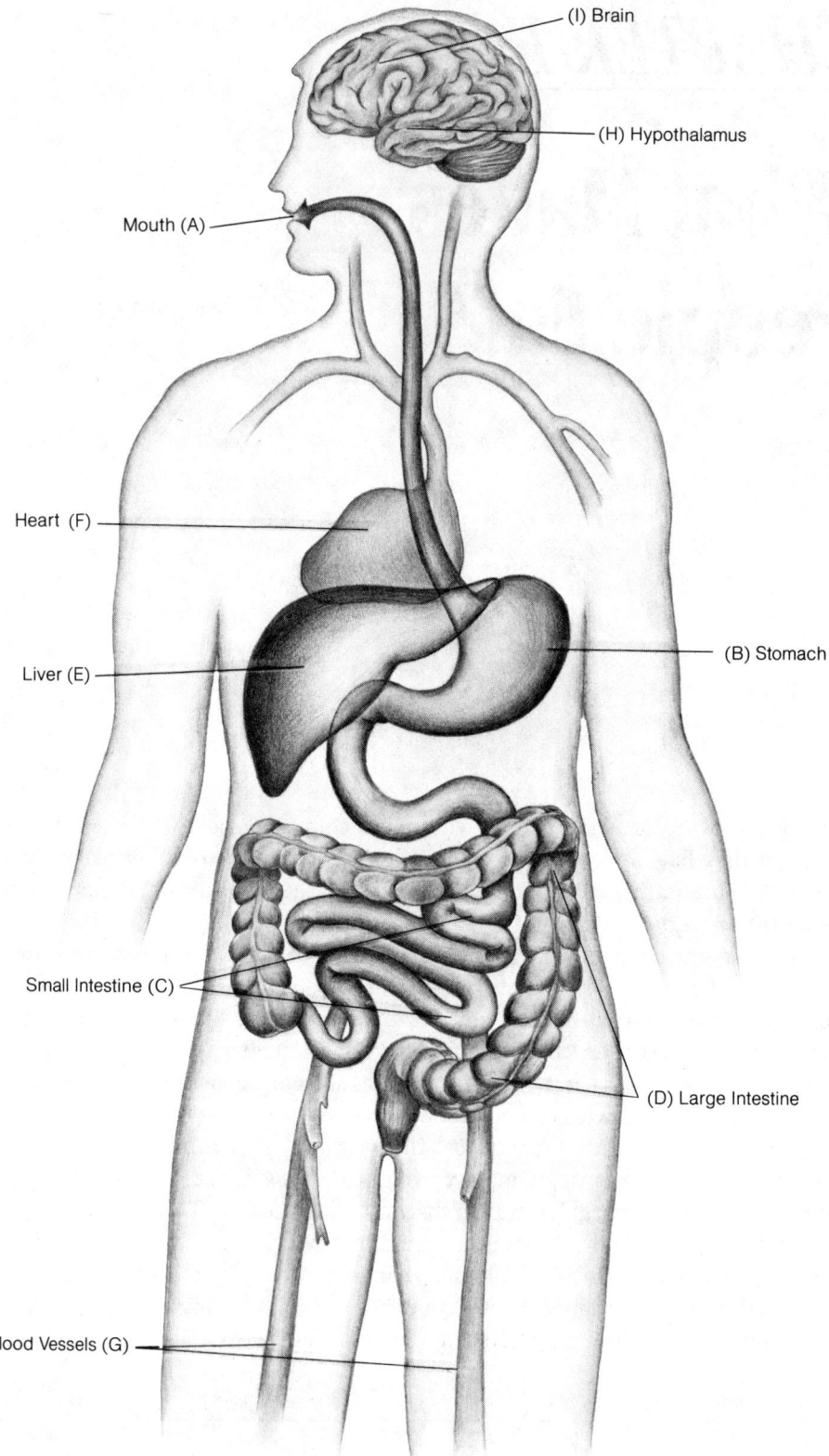

(I) Brain

(H) Hypothalamus

Mouth (A)

Heart (F)

(B) Stomach

Liver (E)

Small Intestine (C)

(D) Large Intestine

Blood Vessels (G)

Fig. 1 Parts of the Human Body That Process Food

and in the systems that regulate the intake, utilization, and storage of food in the body. When the control systems function correctly, normal weight results. When some part of a control system malfunctions, high or low body weight results.

To understand better how control systems work, let us consider briefly how your body utilizes food. Figure 1 is a simplified illustration of your body.

As you chew food in your mouth (A), digestion is started by your saliva. Digestion continues in your stomach (B), and is virtually completed in your small intestines (C). At this point the food is almost completely broken down into small molecules. These small molecules are absorbed by the tiny blood vessels in the walls of your small intestine. The indigestible bulk in your food passes on to your large intestine (D), and is eliminated. The blood flows from the vessels in your small intestine through your liver (E), to your heart (F). From there it is pumped through a system of decreasingly smaller blood vessels (G) to all parts of your body.

In your organs and tissues one of three things happens to the food molecules: (1) they are used to build new tissue, (2) they are used to provide energy for the functions of the body, or (3) they are converted to fat and stored for future use.

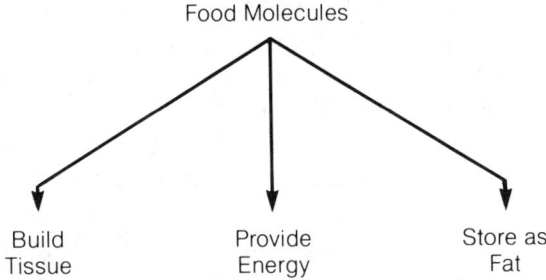

These three processes are known as food *metabolism.* If you eat more food than is needed for new tissue or for energy, your body converts the excess food molecules to fat.

Your body determines how food will be utilized by two types of controls: (1) food intake controls, which regulate the amount of food that gets into your bloodstream; and (2) food metabolism controls, which regulate how the food is used in your body.

Food-Intake Controls

The system that controls the amount of food you eat is found in your hypothalamus (H), a portion of your brain (I), located near the base of the skull.

When one portion of the hypothalamus in a laboratory rat is cut, the animal will not eat even if plenty of food is available. This portion is called the "feeding center." When another portion is cut, the rat will not stop eating until it makes itself grossly overweight. This portion is called the "satiety center." Similar behavior has been found in humans where injuries or tumors have interfered with the function of the hypothalamus.

These centers in the hypothalamus are thought to act like a furnace thermostat and hence are given the name *appestat*. If you set a furnace thermostat at 70 degrees, it will automatically turn on the furnace whenever the room temperature drops below 70 degrees. Then, when the temperature moves just above 70 degrees, the thermostat automatically turns off the furnace.

Your body's appestat is thought to act in a similar manner. There are sensors found in your digestive system, bloodstream, fat storage cells, and other locations that send signals to the appestat that there is, or is not, enough food in your body. When these sensors send "not enough" signals to the appestat, the appestat, in turn, signals "hungry" to your higher brain centers, and you decide to eat. When these sensors send the "enough" signals to the appestat, the appestat signals "full" to your higher brain centers, and you decide to stop eating.

In most persons the appestat works properly to maintain a healthy balance of body weight to height. But in some people the appestat appears to be set too high or too low, and hence gives wrong signals to the higher brain centers. It is like having a defect in your furnace thermostat, which, though set at 70 degrees, keeps the furnace on until the room temperature reaches 85 degrees. An appestat set too high is believed to be the cause of overweight in infants, adolescents, or in adults who suddenly gain much weight. Just as the defective thermostat sends the signal for the furnace to turn on when the room is already hot, so the defective appestat sends genuine "hunger" signals to the higher brain center when the body already has had too much food.

Your body has at least three types of sensors that send signals to the appestat. One type of sensor, which is located in your digestive system, regulates the meal-to-meal intake of food. Another type, which is located in your bloodstream, regulates the day-to-day intake. The third type, believed to be located in your fat-storage cells, seems to regulate the long-term food intake.

The signals from your digestive system depend upon the volume of food present, and upon the length of time the food is in your digestive system. The signals from the sensors in your bloodstream depend upon the concentration of food molecules in your blood.

The signals from the fat-storage cells appear to be controlled by a set-point. Until each fat cell is filled to the set-point, the cells continue to send "not enough" signals to your appestat. In some people it appears that the set-point is too high.

When the person diets and loses weight, the fat-storage cells continue to send "not enough" signals to the appestat until the person regains the fat needed to fill the storage cells to the set-point. It has been found that persons who are overfed, particularly in infancy or adolescence, produce a greater than normal number of fat-storage cells. These persons have a difficult time maintaining a normal body weight when they are adults, since all of the extra fat cells are sending "not enough" signals to the appestat.

Even if your sensors and your appestat are functioning properly, the appestat's signals to the higher brain centers may be overridden by stronger signals from your environment.

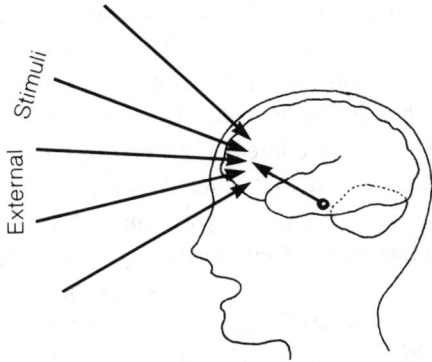

For example, if your parents made you eat all the food on your plate whether you were still hungry or not, you learned that a clean plate was a signal for "full." Or, if you were rewarded for good behavior with an ice cream cone, good behavior became a signal for eating. If you were given candy to compensate for a skinned knee, a hurt became a signal for eating. As you responded to these environmental signals regularly, you developed "eating habits." Perhaps as a teen-ager you found that a box of chocolates compensated for your loneliness on a dateless evening. Loneliness became a signal to eat. Or maybe as an adult you found that a piece of cake was a cure for boredom: boredom became a signal to eat. Or the TV commercial became a signal to eat. Maybe the sight or smell of tasty food supplied a signal. Eventually, responding to these signals developed into very complex and deeply rooted eating habits. You might not even be aware of the habits, but when the proper signal is received, you decide to eat.

Food-Metabolism Controls

As we mentioned earlier, the conversion of food to tissues, energy, or storage fat is known as metabolism. These three processes are very complex, each involving many steps. Each step is controlled by one or more special molecules known as *hormones* and *enzymes*. A defect in the function of any of the hormones or enzymes will interfere with the metabolic step that it controls and may disrupt the whole process.

Two of the best-known hormones are thyroxine and insulin. Thyroxine, a hormone produced by the thyroid gland, is known to affect the metabolism. When the thyroid gland excretes too little thyroxine, the metabolism slows down. That means that less food is converted to new tissue or energy, and more of it is converted to fat; this causes a person to become overweight. Hence some physicians administer thyroid extracts as a part of a weight-control program.

Insulin, a hormone produced by the pancreas, is known to affect the entrance of food molecules into the cells. When too little insulin is produced, in a condition known as diabetes, the cells cannot use the food molecules properly. The opposite condition, too much insulin, often leads to obesity. Research is now being conducted to learn how to control the overproduction of insulin.

Recent research has indicated that other enzyme defects may be involved in obesity. Scientists found that some obese persons have a deficiency of a special enzyme that participates in various energy-using reactions of the body. It is possible that the deficiency of this enzyme might have caused the obesity.

Recent research has discovered another type of metabolic defect that may be a cause of obesity. In normal individuals a type of fat cells known as "brown fat" appear to be able to "waste" energy. When a normal person overeats, the growth of brown fat increases, and the extra food energy is converted to heat and eliminated by radiation or perspiration. Obese persons may have a defect in the brown-fat tissue so that in these individuals the extra calories are converted to fat tissue rather than being wasted as heat.

With hundreds of enzymes and hormones involved in food metabolism, there is a great possibility for a defect in the function of one or more of them. These defects may be hereditary; hence we say that some people have a genetic predisposition to obesity. However, even if you have such a defect, you can still compensate for it by adjusting your diet and life-style.

Activity

Of the three metabolic processes—conversion to new tissue, to energy, or to storage fat—the one most directly related to activity is the one in which food is converted to energy. The body requires energy to carry out all of its functions. For example, energy is required in digestion, in building new tissue, and in causing the brain to function. The single largest use of energy is in the movement of skeletal muscles. If a person's job or life-style restricts the frequent and/or vigorous use of muscles, the body's primary option is to convert the unused energy food to storage fat.

Physical inactivity is believed to be the major cause of "creeping obesity"

—the kind that comes on gradually until you find in middle age that you are overweight. Our modern life seems to conspire to make us inactive. The "good life" is one in which we do not have to work. Inactivity is a symbol of affluence. When we can trade our power mower for a riding lawn mower, we are moving up the success ladder. We have status when an electric machine opens our cans, washes our dishes, disposes of our food wastes, and compacts our trash. We even have a push button for our TV set so we don't have to interrupt our evening of inactivity by getting up to change the channel. And now the ultimate is being developed: Computers that will allow us to sit back and watch the vacuum cleaner or lawn mower being guided around the house or lawn.

But what has this inactivity done to our bodies? The bodies of all animals, including humans, are designed for a certain level of activity. It has been found that below a certain skeletal muscle activity level it is not possible for the body to balance its energy intake and energy expenditure. For example when an animal is confined and not allowed the required activity, the animal becomes fat —witness the "pen-fed" steer or the pampered house pet.

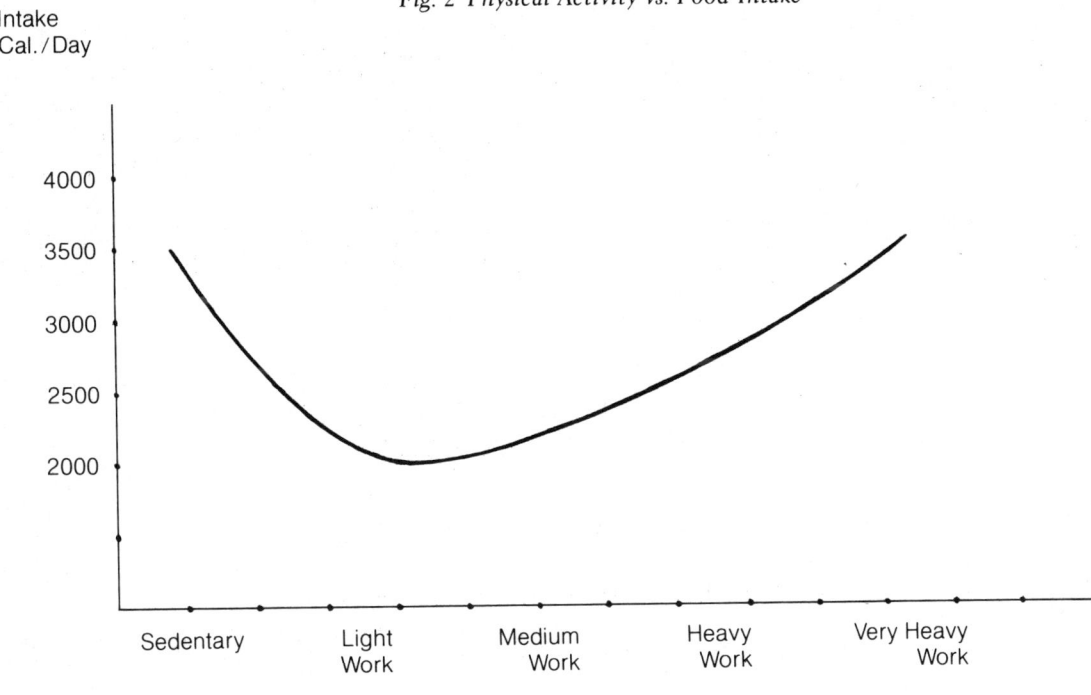

Fig. 2 Physical Activity vs. Food Intake

WHAT MAKES PEOPLE FAT?

Some well-known research suggests that low levels of activity may place people in double jeopardy. Not only does low activity force the body to store unused food as fat, it also increases the appetite. The study showed that, given a choice, people who had moderate activity ate less than people with low activity. Low activity helps you gain weight in two ways: You convert less food to energy, and you eat more food.

Suppose you feel that you are one of those persons trapped by a mis-set control, a metabolic defect, or a life-style over which you feel you have no control. What can you do about it? Is there any hope, or are you doomed to your present dimensions forever?

The general answer lies in the fact that once food has been digested, the body can do only three things with it: (1) convert it to energy, (2) build new tissue, or (3) store it as fat. Therefore, any food not converted to energy or new tissue must be stored as fat. If you wish to make a permanent change in your body weight, you must make permanent changes in the kind and amount of food you eat and in your activity level. Making these changes is not easy. But you will find it easier after you learn some basic information about your body. Then you will understand why, when, and how each effort you make will have the desired effect.

CHAPTER 2

Walking the Tightrope

Your body's balance of nutrients is similar to the balance required of a circus tightrope walker. If she is perfectly balanced, all is well. If she leans a little to one side or other, she can still recover. If she leans too far, she will go crashing to the ground (or to the waiting net). Similarly, your body requires a certain balance of each nutrient. If in one meal you eat too much of one nutrient or too little of another, you can compensate at the next meal or the next day. However, if your nutrients are out of balance for a long time, the situation will be similar to the falling tightrope walker—and your body becomes sick. If you take corrective measures soon enough to restore the nutrient balance, your body can be returned to a state of health.

The absence of any nutrient can be disastrous to your body. But, on the other hand, a great excess of any nutrient is also harmful to your body. The most important factor to consider in planning a long-term diet is the balance among the various nutrients. You must take into account the interrelationships that exist among the nutrients. For example, an excess of one nutrient may hinder the absorption of another nutrient.

There is no one diet that is ideal for everyone, since individuals differ in their requirements for the various nutrients. It *is* possible to chemically analyze your food, blood, tissues, hair, and all your waste products to determine your nutrient status and balance. However the procedure is very costly and is usually done only for research purposes. Instead, guidelines for balanced diets have been established by various organizations in different countries. One guideline was established by the U.S. Senate Select Committee on Nutrition and Human Needs in 1977. This guideline sets up goals for types of foods, such as complex carbohydrates, sugars, kinds of fats, and salt. The Food and Nutrition Board of the National Academy of Sciences–National Research Council has set up dietary standards for nutrients such as vitamins, minerals, and protein for the people of the United States. These standards, which are known as the "Recommended Daily Allowances" (RDAs), have been established after years of research. They are revised every few years as new information becomes available. Standards have been established for protein, for several vitamins and minerals, but not for carbohydrate or fat. The chart below gives the values for some of the RDAs for women and men between twenty-three and fifty years of age.

	Protein G	Vit. A IU	Vit. C MG	Thiamin MG	Ribo. MG	Niacin MG	Vit. B$_6$ MG	Folacin MG	Calcium MG	Iron MG
Woman	44	4000	60	1.0	1.2	13	2.0	0.4	800	18
Man	56	5000	60	1.4	1.6	18	2.2	0.4	800	10

The RDAs are the level of essential nutrients considered by the Food and Nutrition Board to be adequate to meet the known nutritional needs of practically all healthy persons. The RDAs do not take into account special needs arising from infections, metabolic disorders, chronic diseases, or other abnormalities. A copy of the complete 1980 revision of the U.S. RDA is found in Appendix B. Nutritionists use this standard to evaluate an individual's diet. The nutrient information on food labels is also based on this standard. For most processed foods you can determine the percent of your daily needs for each nutrient listed that the food supplies. To evaluate the nutrient composition of unlabeled foods, you can use a table of food composition, such as the one published by the U.S. Department of Agriculture. You can then compare the nutrient content of the food, as obtained from the tables, with the RDAs to evaluate your daily diet. We do not recommend this approach because the task is so complex and time-consuming that it requires a computer to make it convenient. Instead we encourage you to plan a balanced diet using simplified food lists that have been devised by nutritionists (see Chapter 9). First, however, we want you to understand the effects that too much or too little of the various nutrients have on the body.

Water

The most essential nutrient is water. The body cannot survive many days without water. Water transports all nutrients and waste products through the body; water regulates body temperature and salt concentrations. All of the chemical reactions of the body take place in a water solution. Some chemical reactions require water as part of the process.

In healthy persons the body has a fine-tuned water balance controlled by the thirst center, which is located in the hypothalamus near the appestat. The body has no place to store water, so all of the water lost in twenty-four hours must be replaced in that twenty-four hours. Given below is the water balance of an average healthy person.

WATER INTAKE		WATER OUTPUT	
FLUIDS	1250 ml (2.5 pints)	URINE	1400 ml (2.8 pints)
WATER IN FOODS	900 ml (1.8 pints)	FECES	100 ml (0.2 pints)
METABOLIC WATER*	350 ml (0.7 pints)	SKIN	700 ml (1.4 pints)
	2500 ml (5.0 pints)	LUNGS	300 ml (0.6 pints)
			2500 ml (5.0 pints)

*WATER PRODUCED IN BODY CHEMICAL REACTIONS.

Various illnesses upset the water balance. The most important of these are illnesses that are accompanied by vomiting, diarrhea, or bleeding; these may result in life-threatening dehydration. Too much water can be a problem also. For instance, if water is injected into the bloodstream, it can be fatal.

Vitamins

Vitamins are small molecules that are absolutely necessary for many of the metabolic reactions in the body. Unlike some nutrients, vitamins cannot be made by the body and must be supplied in the diet. Outright deficiency of any vitamin results in very serious metabolic malfunctions. Partial deficiencies may result in general symptoms of illness.

Vitamins are classed as *water soluble* or *fat soluble*. The water-soluble vitamins include ascorbic acid (vitamin C), thiamin (vitamin B_1), riboflavin (vitamin B_2), niacin, vitamin B_6, folacin, and vitamin B_{12}. These vitamins are not stored in the body to any extent and must be replenished daily. The fat-soluble vitamins include vitamin A, vitamin D, vitamin E, and vitamin K. These are stored in the liver and need to be replenished only as the stores are used up.

Table 1 Vitamins

Vitamin	Some Functions	Food Sources	Deficiency Symptoms	Symptoms of Excess
Vitamin A	Helps night vision Helps form mucous membranes Helps prevent infection Helps form bone, teeth Promotes growth	Liver, butterfat, egg yolk, apricots, yellow and dark green vegetables	Night blindness, poor growth, infections	Stunted growth, bone fragility, liver disorders in adults
Vitamin D	Helps form bone, teeth	Fish-liver oils, fortified foods	Rickets—poor bone development, osteomalacia —reduced bone minerals	Excessive minerals in lungs, kidneys; headache, nausea
Vitamin E	Protects vitamins A and C Protects cell membranes	Wheat germ oil, nuts, vegetable oils, egg yolk	A type of anemia, muscle weakness, reproductive disorders in animals	Possibly interferes with blood clotting
Thiamin (Vit. B_1)	Coenzyme involved in burning carbohydrates Helps nerve functions Promotes growth	Wheat germ oil, pork, liver, grains, potatoes	Beri-beri—nervous system degeneration, fatigue, deep muscle pain, cardiac failure	None known
Riboflavin (Vit. B_2)	Coenzyme for using oxygen in cells	Milk, dairy products, liver, whole grains, green leafy vegetables	Disorders of skin and eyes	None known
Niacin	Coenzyme for using oxygen in cells, for metabolism	Fish, liver, meat, poultry, grains, eggs, milk, legumes	Pellagra—muscular weakness, nerve, skin disorders, diarrhea	No real toxic effects known
Pyridoxine (Vit. B_6)	Coenzyme for metabolism of amino acids	Liver, milk, whole grains, egg yolk, legumes	A type of anemia, skin disorders, nerve disorders	No real toxic effects known
Folacin	Coenzyme to make DNA	Green leafy vegetables, liver, wheat, eggs, fish	A type of anemia, poor growth, digestive disorders	None known
Vitamin B_{12}	Coenzyme for normal function of metabolism in all cells	Liver, milk, meat, eggs	Pernicious anemia	None known
Ascorbic Acid (Vit. C)	Coenzyme in metabolism of amino acids Helps form teeth and bone Helps heal wounds Helps hold body cells together Helps heal infections Essential to form connective tissue	Citrus fruits, tomatoes, peppers, melons, greens, strawberries	Scurvy—weakness, poor appetite and growth, anemia, swollen gums, swollen wrist and ankle joints, bleeding, depression	Possible kidney stones

Table 1 gives the functions, food sources, symptoms of deficiencies, and symptoms of excesses of most of the vitamins. Only within the last forty years have vitamin-deficiency diseases declined in the United States. However, with the fortifications of food with vitamins A, D, thiamin, riboflavin, niacin, and ascorbic acid, the major deficiency diseases, such as night blindness, rickets, beriberi, pellagra, and scurvy have become rare. The only common vitamin deficiencies at present are vitamin B_{12} deficiencies among strict vegetarians, and folacin deficiencies among pregnant women.

Excesses of vitamins from food are highly unlikely (unless you live on polar-bear liver). However, with the introduction of vitamin supplements excesses sometimes occur. Because water-soluble vitamins are not stored in the body, and the amount not used is excreted, there are no known toxicities from excesses of these vitamins. However, temporary side effects have been reported from large doses of vitamin pills. Doses of 100 mg or more of niacin produce a flushing of the skin and tingling of the limbs. Doses of 100 mg or more of vitamin B_6 have been reported to cause sleepiness in some persons.

Ascorbic acid (vitamin C) is taken in excess more than any other vitamin. After many years of research controversy still exists concerning the value, or danger, of large daily doses. Ascorbic acid appears to be one of the least toxic substances known; many persons have taken doses from 1000 to 10,000 mg per day for many years without ill effects. However, there is some evidence that large doses may cause kidney stones or a temporary rebound scurvy (symptoms of scurvy appear when the doses are discontinued). It is generally accepted that doses of 500 mg a day are safe for most persons.

Since the fat-soluble vitamins can be stored in the body, toxic levels are reached occasionally. Toxic effects of large doses of vitamins A and D have been reported, especially in children. Vitamins E and K are not known to be toxic.

Minerals

The minerals needed by your body in relatively large amounts are calcium, phosphorus, sulfur, potassium, chloride, sodium, and magnesium. Other minerals, known as *trace minerals*, are needed in much smaller amounts. These include iron, fluoride, zinc, copper, iodide, chromium, selenium, manganese, molybdenum, nickel, silicon, and vanadium. The minerals must be supplied in your diet, since your body is not able to make any of them.

Minerals have many different functions in your body. Calcium, phosphorus, magnesium, and fluoride are involved in the structure of your bones and teeth. Sulfur is a component of many proteins, especially those found in hair and nails. Iron is a part of your blood hemoglobin, which transports oxygen from your lungs to your cells. Almost all of the minerals act as cofactors for various

TABLE 2 MINERALS

MINERAL	SOME FUNCTIONS	FOOD SOURCES	DEFICIENCY SYMPTOMS	SYMPTOMS OF EXCESS
CALCIUM	STRUCTURE OF BONES, TEETH; NERVE TRANSMISSION; MUSCLE CONTRACTION; BLOOD CLOTTING; HEARTBEAT REGULATION; COENZYME	MILK, DAIRY PRODUCTS, FISH BONES, SALAD GREENS	RICKETS—ABNORMAL BONE DEVELOPMENT; OSTEOMALACIA—REDUCED BONE MINERALS; OSTEOPOROSIS—REDUCED BONE TISSUE; MUSCLE CRAMPS	NOT LIKELY IN ADULTS
SODIUM	WATER BALANCE, ELECTROLYTE BALANCE	SALT, MOST FOODS EXCEPT FRUITS	SALT DEPLETION, NAUSEA, VOMITING	WATER RETENTION, NAUSEA, VOMITING
POTASSIUM	NEUROMUSCULAR ACTIVITY	FRUITS, MILK, CEREALS, LEGUMES, VEGETABLES	MUSCULAR WEAKNESS, MENTAL APATHY	NOT KNOWN IN ADULTS
IRON	HEMOGLOBIN COENZYME	LIVER, MEAT, EGG YOLK, LEGUMES, WHOLE GRAINS, DARK GREEN VEGETABLES	ANEMIA	NOT KNOWN IN ADULTS
ZINC	PART OF INSULIN COENZYME	MILK, LIVER, SHELLFISH, WHEAT BRAN	POOR GROWTH, POOR WOUND HEALING	NOT KNOWN
IODINE	THYROID HORMONES	IODIZED SALT, SEAFOOD	GOITER	NOT SIGNIFICANT
FLUORIDE	MORE STABLE BONE AND TEETH	DRINKING WATER, RICE, SOYBEANS, ONIONS, SPINACH	DENTAL CARIES, FRAGILE BONES	TEETH MOTTLING
CHROMIUM	GLUCOSE METABOLISM, COENZYME	CORN OIL, MEATS, WHOLE GRAINS, BREWER'S YEAST	POSSIBLY INVOLVED IN DIABETES, HEART DISEASE	NOT KNOWN IN ADULTS

important reactions in your body. Table 2 gives some of the functions, food sources, symptoms of deficiency, and symptoms of excess of several key minerals.

Calcium and iron are the minerals most commonly deficient in the American diet. Persons who do not use milk or dairy products are likely to be deficient in calcium. Although the RDA for calcium can be obtained from four cups of cooked cabbage, spinach, or other greens, very few persons will regularly eat such large amounts. Also most greens contain oxalates—compounds that hinder the absorption of calcium. Middle-aged and older women are most likely to have calcium deficiencies, which result in muscle aches, bone pain, and spontaneous fractures.

Children and women of childbearing age are most likely to have iron deficiency anemia. It is very difficult to obtain the recommended amount of iron each day without an iron supplement. Recent research has shown that vitamin C enhances iron absorption from the intestines. To be effective the vitamin C must be taken at the same meal as the iron-rich food. For example you could drink a glass of orange juice after you eat your breakfast egg. It is especially recommended that children be given vitamin C–rich food with iron-rich food, so that they will be able to obtain enough iron for their needs.

Zinc and chromium deficiency appear to be the result of a diet high in refined grains, such as white rice, bread, and pasta. Almost all minerals are removed from grains when the grains are refined. Zinc deficiency is also found in persons who consume unleavened bread as their major source of food energy. Grains contain a molecule, called *phytate,* which ties up the zinc so that it is poorly absorbed. The enzymes in yeast break down the phytate, thus making the zinc more readily absorbed.

Iodine deficiency, which results in an enlarged thyroid gland, in a condition called *goiter,* was once very common in all inland sections of the U.S. Thanks to the widespread use of iodized salt, this deficiency is now rare. Potassium deficiency sometimes occurs in persons who take diuretics for a long period of time to control hypertension.

All of the minerals are toxic in amounts approximately ten times the RDA. This is usually not a problem with the major minerals such as calcium because the body just will not absorb such large amounts. When it does absorb them, as in the case of sodium and potassium, the kidneys usually eliminate the excess. However, if a person has a kidney malfunction, the excess is not eliminated. Potassium generally is not a problem, but most Americans consume about three times as much sodium (usually as salt) as needed each day. A high salt intake will cause your body to retain water to dilute the extra salt until your kidneys can eliminate it. Persons with a genetic kidney defect are not able to eliminate the extra salt and so retain the water permanently. This retained water increases the blood pressure, resulting in a condition known as *essential hypertension.* Hypertension is a major risk factor in heart disease and stroke.

Since the trace minerals are needed only in very small amounts, it is possible to consume toxic amounts. This usually happens when the drinking water contains a high concentration of the mineral. However, toxic amounts can also be obtained from mineral tablets, especially by children who have been known to eat whole bottles of sugar-coated mineral tablets. In adults there is a mechanism that helps prevent the absorption of excess amounts of some minerals, such as iron; this mechanism is not well developed in infants and children.

Minerals in your body are kept at carefully controlled concentrations in the blood. For example, calcium is required for building bones and teeth, but it is also necessary in your blood for functions such as muscle contraction, nerve transmission, blood clotting, and regulation of your heartbeat. For these vital functions the concentration of calcium in your blood must remain at the necessary level. The level of calcium in your blood is lowered by the following factors: an inadequate intake of dietary calcium; by an inadequate intake of vitamin D, which is required for the absorption and utilization of calcium; by an excess of dietary phosphorus such as found in soft drinks, which interferes with the absorption and utilization of calcium; by very high protein diets (about two times the RDA); and by a lack of physical activity. If insufficient calcium is supplied to the blood, it will take calcium from your bones. A prolonged deficiency of calcium in your blood will result in porous and fragile bones.

Proteins

A daily intake of protein is necessary to supply the amino acids to rebuild your body's tissues. In addition to getting enough protein, it is also important to eat protein containing the right kind of amino acids. Of the twenty amino acids required by the body, eight of them (nine for children) are called "essential" because your body cannot make them from other amino acids. Foods that contain the right proportions of the essential amino acids are known as "complete" protein foods. Milk and eggs are considered the best of the complete protein foods, but meat, poultry, and fish are also very good. Most plant protein foods, such as grains, nuts, and legumes (dried peas and beans) are considered "incomplete" protein foods.

Incomplete protein foods can be a good dietary source of protein in combination with complementary foods. Complementary combinations are those that combine a food low in amino acid no. 1, but high in amino acid no. 2, with a food low in no. 2, but high in no. 1. Grains and legumes, nuts and legumes, or dairy products and grains are complementary combinations. The following list shows some complementary protein combinations.

TACO – CORN, BEEF, CHEESE

RICE AND TOFU – SOYBEAN CURD, RICE

BURRITO – CORN, BEANS

MIXED NUTS

FISH AND POI

BREAD AND MILK

Protein deficiency is most disastrous to a developing fetus. If the fetus does not die, the child will usually be born with brain damage. In infants and small children a protein deficiency causes brain damage and lack of growth. Protein deficiency in adults primarily causes muscle wasting.

Protein excess can also be damaging to the body. Extra amino acids will be converted to fat (on a diet adequate in carbohydrate and fat), or burned as energy (on a diet low in carbohydrate and fat), or converted to glucose (on a low-carbohydrate diet). However, in each of these conversions there remains a nitrogen waste product that must be eliminated by the kidneys. If the kidneys cannot handle the overload, some of the waste products may lead to a condition known as gout. The overload may itself damage the kidneys. In addition if there is not enough glucose available to help convert the protein to energy, some of the amino acids will be converted to substances known as *ketone bodies*. The presence of ketone bodies in the blood results in a clinical condition known as *ketosis*. Some of the symptoms of this condition are "acetone breath," headaches, and fatigue; severe ketosis will cause coma.

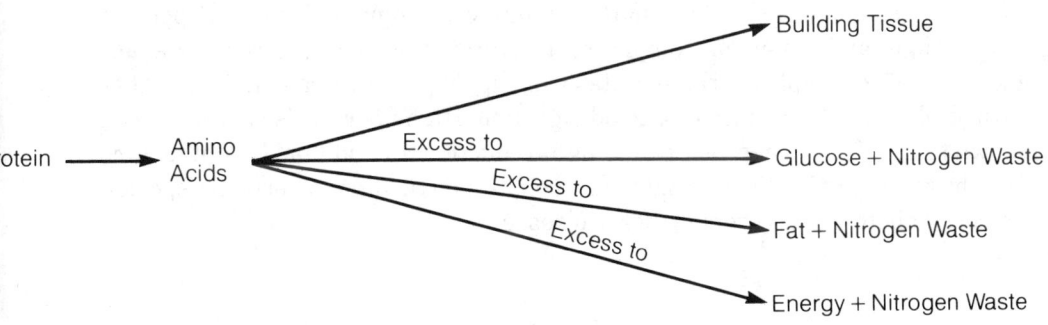

Carbohydrates

Carbohydrates, which are broken down in the digestive system to simple sugars, are used primarily for energy, although small amounts are used to build parts of certain tissues. Brain and certain other tissues must use glucose for energy, so a deficiency in dietary carbohydrates results in dietary protein and

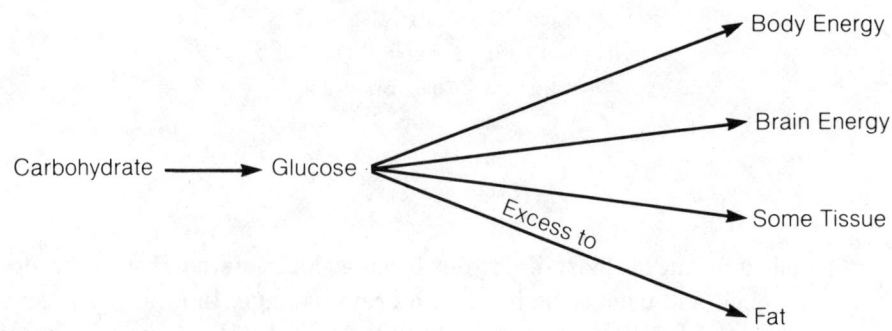

your own muscle protein being used for energy. Excess glucose is converted to fat and stored in the adipose cells.

Carbohydrate can be eaten as complex carbohydrates, such as those found in grains, vegetables, and fruits, or as simple carbohydrates, such as the refined sugars found in table sugar, candies, and other "sweets." All carbohydrates are good food and will provide energy for your body. However, refined sugars provide only energy, since they do not contain vitamins, minerals, or fiber. If the sugars are eaten instead of complex carbohydrates, the person will be deficient in certain vitamins, minerals, and in fiber. If the sugars are eaten in addition to complex carbohydrates, the person will have excess glucose, which will be converted to fat.

At present the American diet contains about 18 percent refined sugar. It has been recommended by the Senate Committee that our diet contain 10 percent refined sugar and 48 percent complex carbohydrates, such as grains, vegetables, and fruits. The complex carbohydrates will supply vitamins, minerals, and fiber to the body. Fiber is required for good digestion. High fiber foods have also been shown to be effective in promoting weight reduction. In addition, lack of dietary fiber has been implicated in conditions such as constipation, diverticulitis, colon cancer, diabetes, and coronary heart disease.

Fats

Fats are broken down in the digestive system to fatty acids. These are used primarily for energy. Certain parts of some tissues also require fatty acids. Those fatty acids not used for tissues or for energy are converted to fat and stored in the adipose cells. Of all the nutrients a high-fat diet has the highest correlation with obesity. Most Americans have a diet that is 40 to 50 percent fat, whereas a diet containing 30 percent fat is recommended by the Senate Committee for good health.

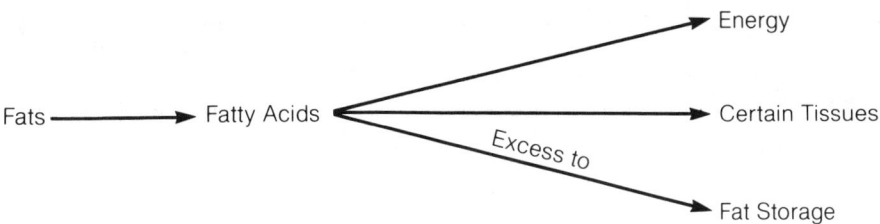

Dietary fats, when digested, produce three kinds of fatty acids: polyunsaturated, monounsaturated, and saturated. Cooking fats that contain mostly saturated fatty acids are solid at room temperature; if they contain mostly unsaturated fatty acids, they are liquid at room temperature. Animal fats contain mostly saturated fatty acids; plant oils, except coconut and palm, contain mostly monounsaturated and polyunsaturated fatty acids.

The significance of the type of fatty acids in the diet is yet to be conclusively determined. The lesions or "plaques" that plug up the arteries in atherosclerosis and lead to heart disease contain mostly cholesterol and saturated fatty acids. In the bloodstream fatty acids and cholesterol are combined with protein in a unit known as *lipoproteins*. There are two main types of lipoproteins: high-density lipoproteins (HDL), which carry about 25 percent of the cholesterol in the blood, and low-density lipoproteins (LDL), which carry more than 70 percent of the circulating cholesterol. High blood levels of HDL seem to prevent heart disease, whereas high levels of LDL are the most important risk factor in heart disease. There is some evidence that the LDL carry the cholesterol *to* the cells, and the HDL carry the cholesterol *away from* the cells.

Factors that increase the LDL blood level are cigarette smoking, obesity, high consumption of cholesterol and saturated fats, and most types of oral contraceptives. Factors that increase the HDL blood level are a diet high in vegetables, grains, fish with very little meat or processed fats, and certain plant fibers, such as pectin, but not bran; and high physical activity. Whole milk, in contrast to other foods containing saturated fats, does not raise the LDL level, but may even lower the level (thought to be due to the high calcium content of milk). Moderate amounts of eggs (up to one per day) seem not to raise the LDL levels. Dietary polyunsaturated fatty acids reduce the LDL level in some persons. Women, before the menopause, have higher HDL levels than men.

The best dietary recommendations for the prevention of heart disease that can be given at present are (1) stop, or do not start, smoking; (2) attain and maintain your ideal weight; (3) lower your consumption of animal and hydrogenated vegetable fats; (4) replace some of your saturated fats with unsaturated fats; (5) increase your consumption of fruits, vegetables, and grains; (6) drink milk or use in cooking; and (7) limit yourself to one egg per day.

TABLE 3   BALANCE OF PROTEIN, CARBOHYDRATES, AND FATS

TYPE OF NUTRIENTS	% OF TOTAL DAILY CALORIES
PROTEIN (SUCH AS MEAT, EGGS, CHEESE, DRIED BEANS)	12–15
COMPLEX CARBOHYDRATES (SUCH AS GRAINS, VEGETABLES, FRUIT)	45–48
REFINED SUGARS (SUCH AS SUGAR, HONEY, CANDY)	10
SATURATED FATS (SUCH AS BUTTER, BACON, EGG YOLK, SOLID MARGARINES)	10
POLYUNSATURATED FATS (SUCH AS CORN, SOYBEAN, SUNFLOWER, SAFFLOWER OILS)	10
MONOUNSATURATED FATS (SUCH AS PEANUT OIL AND PEANUT BUTTER)	10

FOR AN AVERAGE 154-LB. MALE OR AN AVERAGE 120-LB. FEMALE,
THE ABOVE TABLE TRANSLATES TO THE FOLLOWING:

TYPE OF NUTRIENT	MALE		FEMALE	
	GRAMS	KITCHEN MEASURE	GRAMS	KITCHEN MEASURE
COMPLEX CARBOHYDRATES	277	10 OZ.	187	7 OZ.
REFINED SUGARS	58	12 TSP.	39	8 TSP.
SATURATED FATS	26	2 TB.	17	1 TB.
POLYUNSATURATED FATS	26	2 TB.	17	1 TB.
MONOUNSATURATED FATS	26	2 TB.	17	1 TB.
PROTEIN*	63	9 OZ. MEAT	49	7 OZ. MEAT

*Most protein foods are not 100 percent protein. This table assumes 1 oz. meat contains 7 grams protein.

Source: U. S. Senate Select Committee on Nutrition and Human Needs, *Dietary Goals for the United States*, 2nd Ed. Washington, D.C.: U.S. GPO, 1977.

Certain types of cancers are associated with a high-fat diet. Population studies implicate saturated fats; but certain animal studies have also implicated polyunsaturated fats in the formation of certain tumors. However, recent studies suggest that it may be that only hydrogenated polyunsaturates are involved in tumor formation. The best recommendations that can be given at present with regard to fats and cancer are (1) lower your total fat consumption, (2) lower your consumption of hydrogenated oils, (3) avoid cooking in oils that are heated to a high temperature; especially avoid deep-fat frying in oil that has been repeatedly heated.

The recommended proportion of carbohydrates, protein, and fats in our diet is shown in Table 3. The quantity of each of these nutrients that our diet should contain is also given.

CHAPTER 3

Meat Pies to Muscles

How is a drink of milk converted to muscle tissue? How do tortillas and beans become part of nerve cells? How does a bedtime piece of pie become stored fat? How are apples converted to energy? When you understand how the body makes these conversions, you will better understand what you can do to make your food end up as new tissue or energy, rather than as fat. Let us follow the nutrients in a meat pie through your body to see how part becomes new muscle, part becomes energy to power the muscle, and part may be stored as fat.

Digestion

When the meat pie enters your mouth, you begin a process called *digestion*, in which food is broken down into small molecules. As you chew the meat pie, your teeth break up the large pieces into small pieces; but these small pieces still contain billions of large molecules. The digestive enzymes in your saliva help reduce these by breaking down some of the large carbohydrate molecules into smaller molecules.

These smaller molecules, with the rest of the meat pie ingredients, fall down into your stomach, stimulating the production of additional digestive enzymes. In your stomach some protein molecules are broken into smaller fragments. Your stomach churns the partially digested meat pie around for several minutes before passing it on to your small intestine. In your small intestine new enzymes are added that complete the digestive process. The carbohydrates end up as simple sugar molecules, such as glucose. The protein fragments end up as amino acid molecules, and part of the fats as fatty-acid molecules. The vitamins, minerals, and water already exist as small molecules and do not have to be broken down in your digestive system. The fiber molecules are not digested, but are passed into your large intestine, gathering up bacteria and other waste products, and are eliminated.

Figure 3 summarizes the fate of each of the nutrients in the digestive system.

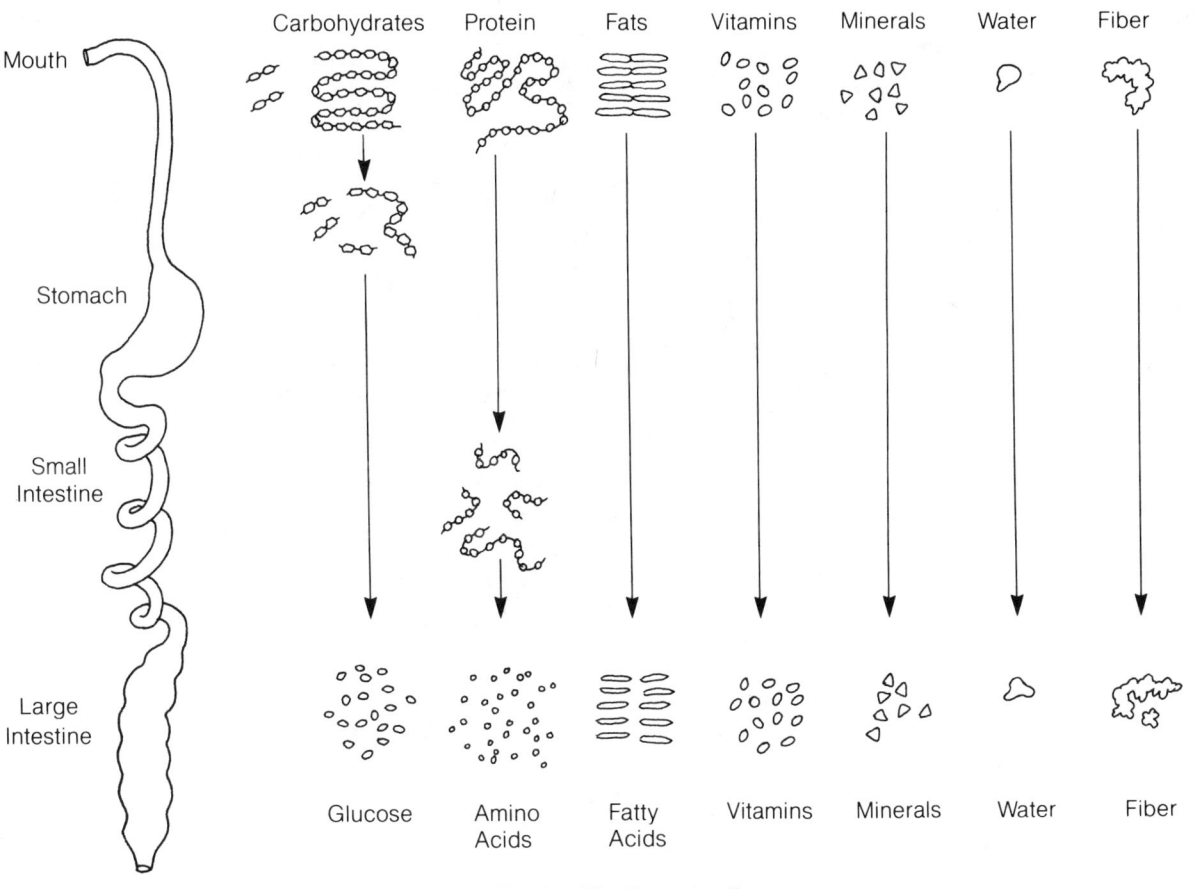

Fig. 3   The Digestive Process

Flow of Nutrients Inside Your Body

The glucose, amino acids, fatty acids, vitamins, minerals, and water from your meat pie pass through the walls of your small intestine into your bloodstream. Let us follow the flow of these nutrients using Figure 4. The molecules are carried by a vein to your liver (A). Some of the nutrient molecules remain in your liver, some are modified and then put back into your bloodstream, and some are sent on unchanged. The blood then carries the nutrient molecules to your heart (B). Your heart is a muscle designed for pumping blood throughout your body. In the trip around your body the blood is first pumped to your lungs (C) to pick up oxygen from the air you breathe, and to release the waste product, carbon dioxide. The blood, now containing both nutrient molecules and oxygen,

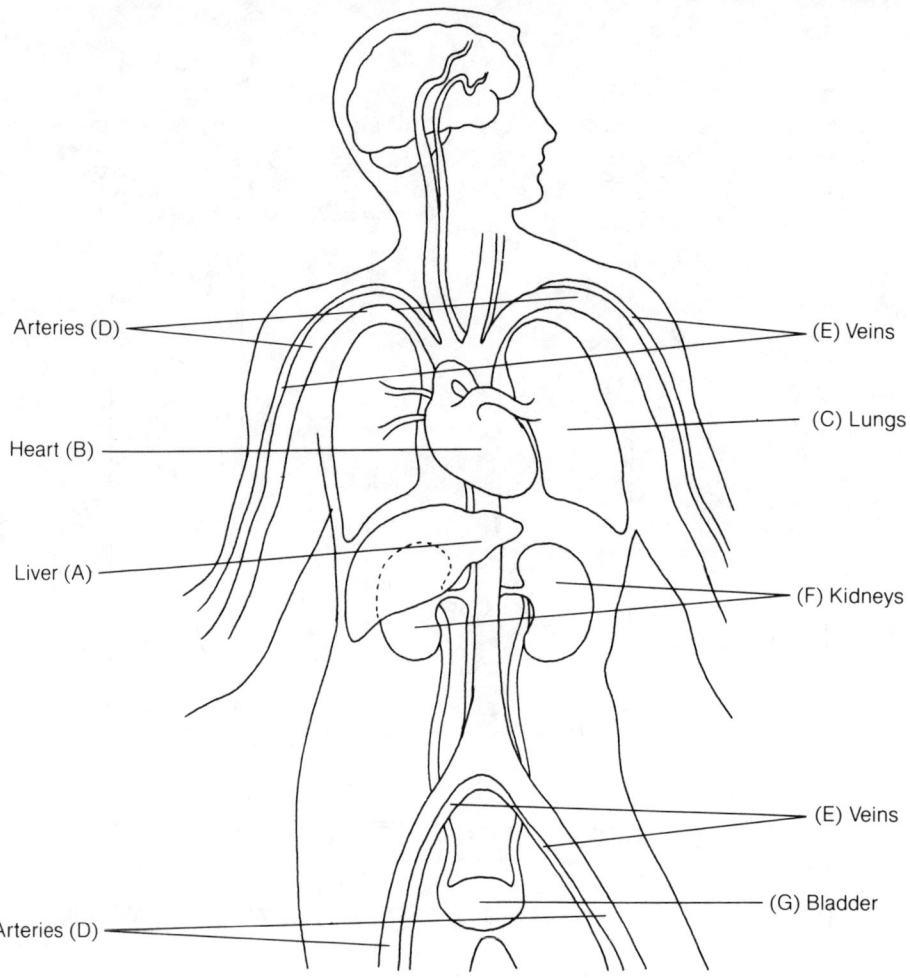

Fig. 4   Flow of Nutrients Inside Your Body

THE BIO-PLAN FOR LIFELONG WEIGHT CONTROL

is then sent to the trillions of cells in your body through a complex system of blood vessels called arteries (D) and capillaries. After the nutrients are used by the cells, the blood carries the waste products back to the heart in vessels called veins (F). During each trip around your body some of the blood containing waste products is sent to your kidneys (G). As the blood flows through your kidneys, the waste products are filtered out and passed to your bladder (H) for elimination.

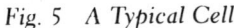

Fig. 5   A Typical Cell

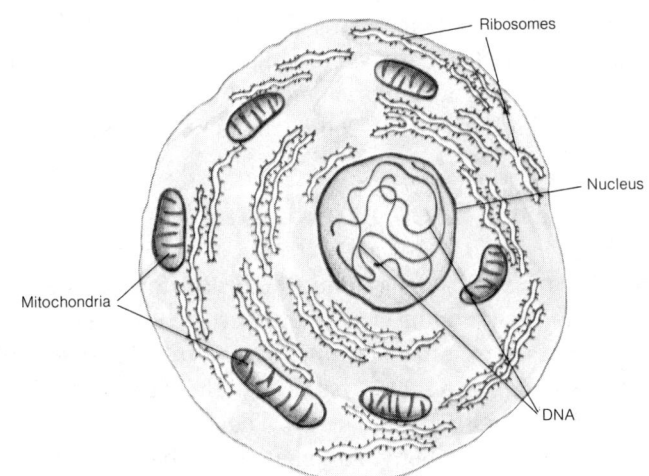

The Cell

The nutrient molecules from your meat pie, along with the oxygen from your lungs, are used in the trillions of cells in all parts of your body. All of the metabolism of nutrient molecules takes place in various compartments of your cells. Figure 5 shows a typical cell with some of its special compartments.

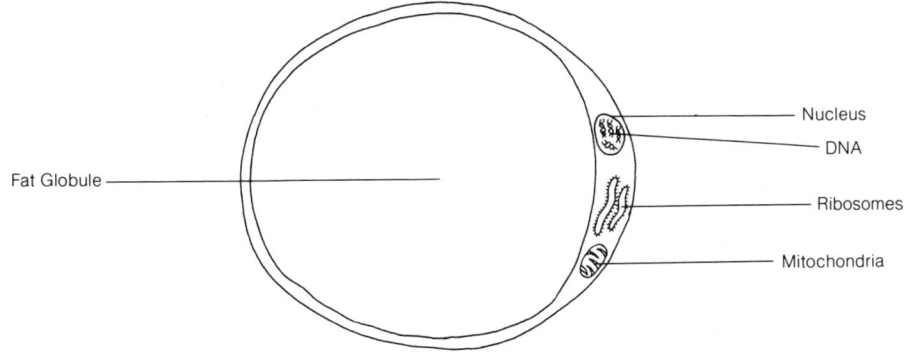

Fig. 6   Adipose Cell

Your chromosomes and genes, which are composed of a special molecule called *DNA*, are found in the *nucleus* of the cell. The DNA is the master controller of the cell. It controls cell division, which makes new cells. It also determines what kind of building materials will be made by the cell from the nutrient molecules. The *ribosomes* are the factories where new proteins are manufactured. The *mitochondria* are the powerhouses where the nutrient molecules are "burned" to provide energy.

Your body also has special cells known as *adipose* cells, which are designed for storing fat. Most adipose cells are found just beneath the skin, although some are associated with most types of tissue. Figure 6 gives a sketch of a typical adipose cell. The big difference between an adipose cell and the "typical" cell is that the nucleus, ribosomes, and mitochondria in the adipose cell are pushed against one wall and the bulk of the cell consists of a globule of fat.

Enzymes and Cofactors

Just as digestive enzymes are required to break down large nutrient molecules, so other enzymes are required to manufacture new tissue molecules and to convert nutrient molecules into energy or storage fat. Enzymes make nutrient molecules react by holding the molecules in just the right position for them to bond to each other, forming larger molecules. There is a specific enzyme for each reaction that takes place in the body. An enzyme can be compared to a lock and the nutrient molecule to a key. The right lock is necessary for the right key.

Many of the enzyme reactions in the cell require a helper molecule, called a *cofactor*. Sometimes the cofactor changes the shape of the enzyme to make it fit the nutrient molecule. This is known as activating the enzyme (see Figure

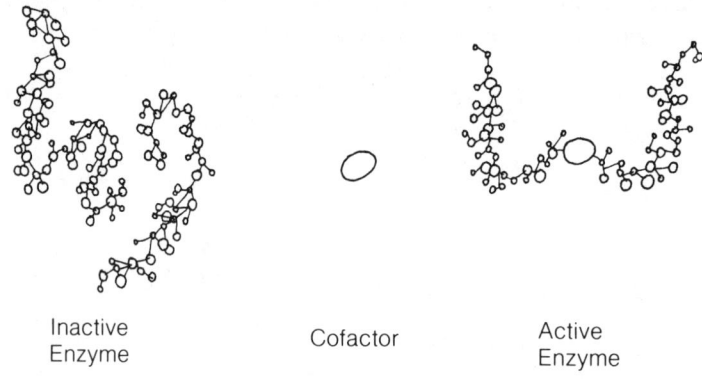

Inactive
Enzyme

Cofactor

Active
Enzyme

Fig. 7   Activation of an Enzyme by a Cofactor

7). Other cofactors are necessary to combine with part of the nutrient molecule to change that molecule into a different one. Vitamins and minerals often act as cofactors. This is one reason vitamins and minerals are essential to your body. If the vitamin or mineral required as a cofactor is not present in the cell, the enzyme reaction cannot take place and new tissue cannot be formed.

Cellular Conversion of Nutrients to New Tissue

Most of the building materials of your body, as well as all the enzymes, are composed of proteins. Your body must build all of its own proteins; you cannot

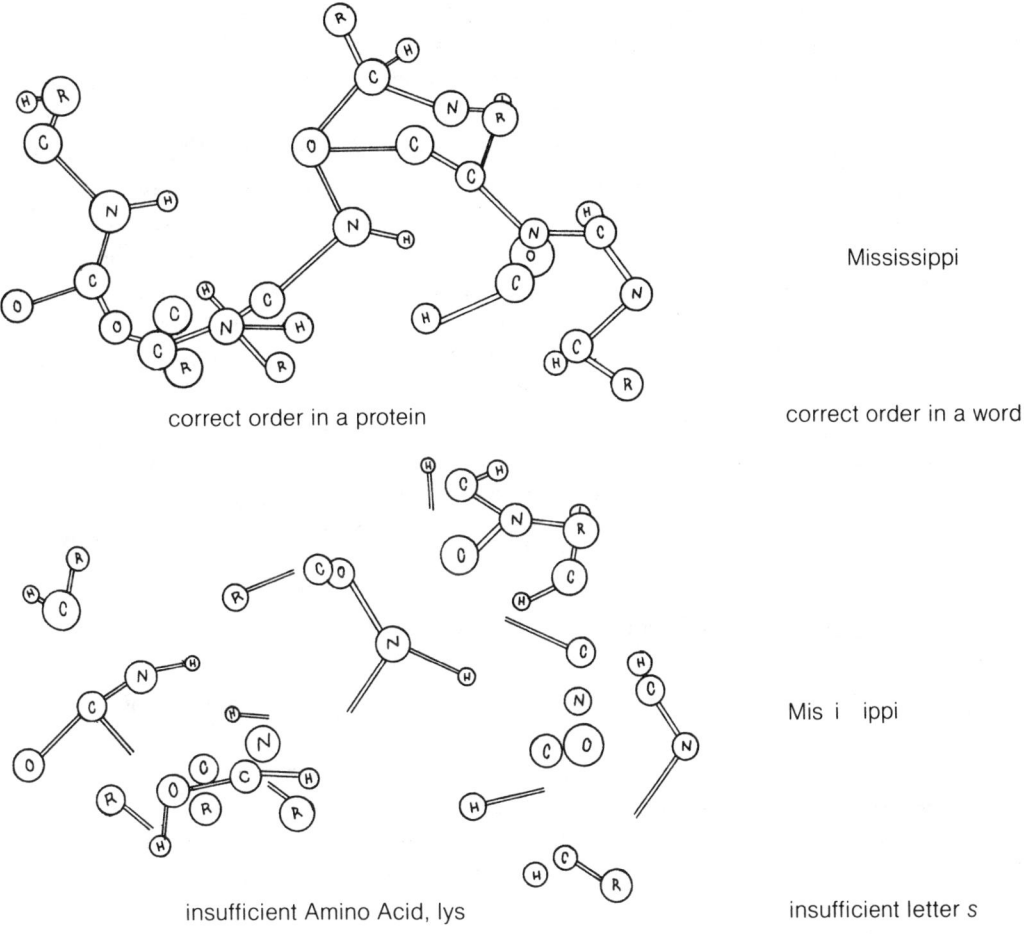

correct order in a protein

Mississippi

correct order in a word

insufficient Amino Acid, lys

Mis i   ippi

insufficient letter *s*

Fig. 8   *Structure of Proteins Compared to Structure of Words*

use the protein from anything else. Hence the most important reason for you to eat the meat pie is to provide amino acids for your cells to use in making your proteins.

Each of the protein molecules in your body is composed of amino acids linked together in a unique order. Building a protein molecule can be considered similar to building a word. If the letters in a word are not in the right order, you won't have the right word. Similarly all the amino acids must be in the correct order in each protein chain.

Your body cells can build the needed protein molecules only if all the required amino acids are contained in the food you eat. If a certain amino acid is present in too small an amount to make the whole protein, that protein cannot be built (just as you cannot build the word *Mississippi* with just one *s*).

One of the strengths of a balanced diet is that it provides the necessary balance of amino acids to build your body proteins.

The construction of proteins also requires energy. Your body is very versatile here. If there is not enough energy available from sugars and fatty acids, your body will use part of the available amino acids as a source of energy. And if there are not enough amino acids available in your food to use as raw materials and energy for building the most critical proteins, your body will break down your own muscle tissue to obtain the necessary amino acids. This is the process that occurs during starvation that results in skeletonlike victims.

Most of the new tissue manufactured in your cells is composed of protein. However, there are some tissues that also require molecules of fatty acids or sugars or minerals for their structure. For example, cell membranes and the insulating sheaths on nerve cells require fatty acids. Sugars are part of the structure of the lubricant found in the joints between your bones. And of course minerals are required for building bones and teeth. Some of the fats or sugar or calcium and phosphorus in your meat pie may be used for these tissues.

Cellular Conversion of Nutrients to Energy

Most of the glucose and fatty-acid molecules from your meat pie are used for energy—provided your body can use the energy (for example, if you consumed the meat pie right before or after a good game of tennis). The conversion of nutrients to energy is a multistep process that requires a specific enzyme and usually a cofactor for each step. The enzymes needed to convert fatty acids to energy are called, by some authors, "fat-burning" enzymes. Figure 9 summarizes the conversion process.

There are two types of conversion of nutrients to energy: (1) *aerobic*, which requires a lot of oxygen, and (2) *anaerobic*, which requires only a small amount of oxygen. Aerobic processes can burn molecules of glucose, fatty acids, or

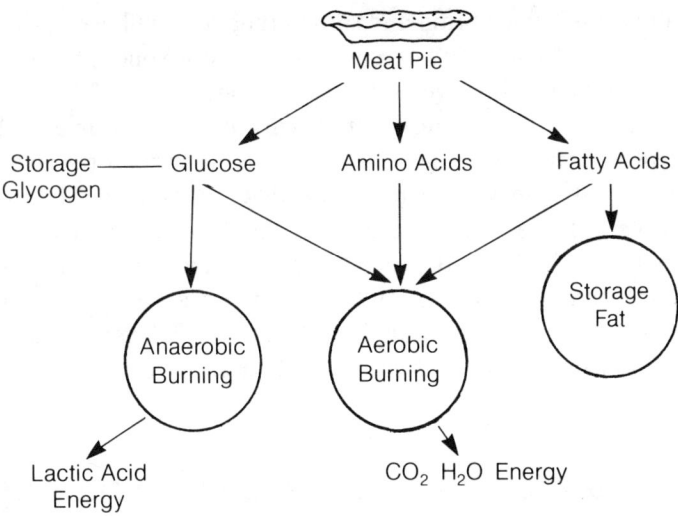

Fig. 9   *Cellular Conversion of Nutrients to Energy*

amino acids, and produce carbon dioxide and water as waste products. Anaerobic processes can burn only glucose molecules, and produce as a waste product a molecule called *lactic acid*. This lactic acid enters your bloodstream and makes the blood more acid, giving you a feeling of fatigue and achy muscles.

Your muscle cells, during light to moderate exercise, use mostly fatty acids in aerobic burning. However, during very strenuous exercise when you are at the point of breathlessness, your muscle cells must burn glucose anaerobically, because there is not enough oxygen present for aerobic burning.

During sustained exercise the nutrients in your bloodstream are quickly used up. The muscle cells then draw on two reservoirs of energy: (1) fat stored in the adipose cells, and (2) glucose stored in the muscle cells in the form of large molecules called *glycogen*. When your muscle activity is prolonged, the fatty acids are withdrawn from the adipose cells, sent to the muscle cells, and burned aerobically for energy. When muscle activity is prolonged and strenuous, the glycogen molecules are broken down into glucose molecules, which are burned anaerobically. When your muscle glycogen stores are depleted, you collapse with exhaustion. You must rest until you obtain sufficient oxygen for the aerobic burning of your fatty acids, and for the conversion of lactic acid back to glucose.

Some cells, such as those in your brain and nerve tissue and your blood cells, can burn only glucose for energy. When you eat carbohydrates, the liver converts much of the glucose to glycogen and stores it for emergency use by these particular cells. Between meals and during periods when you do not eat enough carbohydrates, your brain and these other cells will use up the glycogen supply in your liver. The average person is able to store enough glycogen in the liver to last these tissues for twelve to twenty-four hours. If you go for a few days without eating any, or enough, carbohydrates, your brain and these other tissues must obtain their glucose from a source other than the liver glycogen stores. Unfortunately (for weight reducers) fatty acids cannot be converted to glucose. However, glucose can be made from some of the amino acids. So if you do not eat enough carbohydrate, your body will take these amino acids away from the protein-building processes and use them to make the necessary glucose. Even with adequate protein in your diet, if you are deficient in carbohydrate, your body will break down some of your muscle tissue to convert the amino acids to glucose.

Cellular Conversion of Nutrients to Storage Fat

Storage fats are manufactured in the adipose cells from fatty acids and a molecule derived from glucose. The fatty acids usually come from foods containing fats. However, glucose or amino acids from your food can also be converted to fatty-acid molecules. So if you consume too much of any of these three nutrients, the excess will be converted to fat. Thus if you eat your meat pie after a big meal, the molecules of glucose and fatty acids, and perhaps also the amino acids, will be converted to storage fat.

Once the fat is deposited in the adipose cells, it remains stored until other cells of your body have a need for the energy. For example, assume that the day after you eat the meat pie you enter an athletic event and are injured. You need extra energy for the athletic event and then need extra energy to repair the injured tissue. Now some fats in your adipose cells are broken down into fatty acids by enzymes that some writers call "fat-mobilizing" enzymes. The free fatty acids are then sent to the muscle and the injured tissue cells to be burned to provide energy for muscle motion and for building new proteins to repair the injured tissue.

CHAPTER 4

The Triple Bonus

How would you like a magic pill that would make your body use up your excess fat while you slept? Well, we can't quite give you that, but we can suggest something just about as good. This is the triple bonus you will obtain from increased physical activity.

Energy Expenditure

Almost all foods can be converted, in part, to energy. Food energy is measured in a unit called the *kilocalorie; calorie* for short. A calorie is the amount of heat energy that could be obtained by burning a certain quantity of food completely to carbon dioxide and water. "Calorie counter" tables list this value of heat energy for various foods. As we explained earlier, energy is necessary for your body to carry out all of its functions. Some of these functions, such as brain energy, are so important that if you do not provide enough food energy, your body will break down its own tissues to obtain fuel to provide this energy.

Your body uses up energy even while you are resting or sleeping to carry out its vital functions. This energy is called your *internal energy* and is known as your *basal metabolic energy,* or *basal metabolic rate* (BMR). You do not have much voluntary control over this internal energy; mostly it is a function of your age and sex. Figure 10 shows the average BMR for each sex as a function of age. You will note that the BMR is very high in children, since they require much energy for manufacturing new tissue. You will also note that the BMR continues to decrease each year after you become an adult. This is one reason why you become fat if you eat the same amount of food at age forty as you did at age twenty. The basal metabolic energy for an average adult woman varies from 1200 to 1450 calories per day and from 1600 to 1800 calories for an average

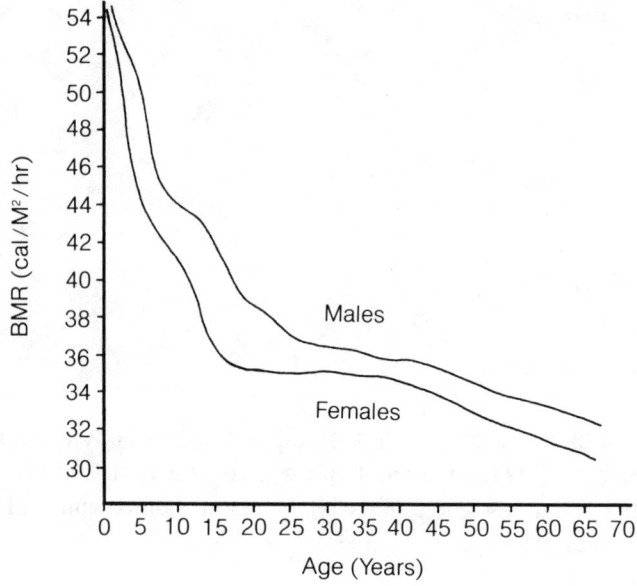

Fig. 10   BMR as a Function of Age

Table 4   *Percent of BMR Used by Various Tissues*

Tissue	% of BMR
Liver	25–28
Brain	19–21
Heart	9–11
Kidneys	7–8
Resting Muscle	25–28
All Other	4–15

adult man. You will note that your liver requires about one quarter of your internal energy. Your liver is the principal manufacturing plant in your body and requires a significant amount of energy for its building processes. Your brain is the master computer for your body and needs energy to control all your body processes. Of course your heart must have energy to pump your blood throughout your body. And your kidneys require energy to filter out the wastes from your blood. A very interesting fact is the high amount of energy required by resting muscle, just to maintain muscle tone. The more muscle tissue you have, the more energy is required for this function. The main reason adult men have a higher BMR than adult women is that a higher percent of a man's body is composed of muscle.

If you are an average sedentary person, your BMR accounts for about two thirds of your daily energy needs; your physical activity accounts for most of the other one third. Of the two, however, physical activity is the only one that you can voluntarily increase. In very active persons physical activity energy may be increased to 50 percent or more of their total daily energy needs. This possibility leads us to consider your first bonus.

Bonus #1

Unlike your BMR, your level of physical activity is something that you can voluntarily control. Different physical activities require different amounts of energy. Table 5 gives examples of the energy requirements of a few types of activities for persons of different body weights. A more complete table is found in Appendix B.

TABLE 5 CALORIE EXPENDITURE PER MINUTE FOR VARIOUS ACTIVITIES

ACTIVITY	125-LB. PERSON	150-LB. PERSON	175-LB. PERSON
	CAL./MIN.	CAL./MIN.	CAL./MIN.
WALKING, 2 MPH	2.9	3.5	4.2
WALKING, 4.5 MPH	5.5	6.7	7.8
BICYCLING, 5.5 MPH	4.2	5.1	5.9
RUNNING, 5.5 MPH	9.0	10.8	12.7

It may seem that the amount of energy used by a physical activity is too small to matter. After all, you have to bicycle rapidly for twenty minutes just to use up 100 calories—the amount found in a large apple. To use up the calories in a piece of pie it would take nearly an hour and a half of bicycling. However, the important point here is that the increased physical activity does not have to be performed all at once. For example, suppose you kept your diet the same, but merely increased your physical activity to include an extra thirty minutes of brisk walking five times a week, every week for a year. The thirty minutes of walking is equivalent to about 150 calories per day or 39,150 calories per year. This is equivalent to a loss of 11.2 pounds in a year without restricting your diet at all. (Actually you will lose 11.2 pounds of fat; your net weight change may be less than that, since some of the fat will be replaced by muscle tissue. Even if your weight loss is not great, your shape will surely improve.)

There are many ways that you can increase your daily activity without even making a special time for exercise or a walk:

1. Get off at an earlier bus stop and walk the last distance to work.
2. Use the stairs rather than the elevator or escalator.
3. Park at the end of the supermarket lot, rather than near the door.
4. Walk to the neighborhood store rather than drive.
5. Go after items yourself rather than sending children for them.
6. Stand up to do your ironing, rather than sitting down.
7. Use a manual, rather than an electric, typewriter.
8. Go after your own supplies, rather than sending your secretary.
9. Take a walk, rather than a doughnut, for your coffee break.
10. Open cans with a manual can opener.
11. Use manual instead of power tools and kitchen appliances.
12. Hang up your clothes to dry rather than using a dryer.
13. Ride a bicycle to work.
14. Walk your dog instead of giving the task to your children.
15. Begin a garden and work in it regularly.

Suppose you decide to increase your physical activity by the following: walking to the neighborhood store, rather than driving; mowing your lawn with a push mower; walking from one end of the shopping center to the other, rather than riding; walking upstairs for items an extra five minutes each day; working in your garden; and standing up to iron rather than sitting down. Table 6 summarizes your extra activity in terms of pounds per year of fat that you will lose with this extra activity.

TABLE 6 POUNDS OF FAT LOST BY INCREASING DAILY ACTIVITY

ACTIVITY	MIN./YEAR	CAL./MIN.	CAL./YR.	LB. LOST/YEAR
WALK TO NEIGHBORHOOD STORE, 10 MIN., 5 TIMES EACH WEEK	2600	3.5	9100	2.6
MOW LAWN WITH PUSH MOWER, 30 MIN./WEEK	1560	5.0	7800	2.2
WALK UPSTAIRS, 5 MIN./DAY EXTRA	1825	6.0	10950	3.1
WALK AT SHOPPING CENTER, 15 MIN./WEEK	780	3.5	2730	0.8
WORK IN GARDEN, 10 MIN., 4 TIMES/WEEK	2080	4.0	8320	2.4
STAND UP TO IRON, 1 1/2 HRS./WEEK	4680	2.0	9360	2.7
TOTAL				13.8 LB.

The small energy increases given in the above example will lead to a loss of 13.8 pounds of fat in a year. This is not a small amount, especially if you continue it from year to year. Thus even though your style of living might not accommodate a vigorous exercise program, you can still make a number of small changes that will develop into habits that permanently increase the energy expenditure of your daily living. Not only will your increased physical activity use up some of your excess fat stores, but the increased amount of muscle in your body will use up extra calories while you are resting or sleeping too. This is your second bonus.

Bonus #2

Most of us markedly decrease our physical activity as we grow older. As our energy expenditure decreases, several things happen to our body. One important result is that our unused muscle tissue atrophies and is replaced by fat tissue. This is known as "fat marbling." To realize just what happens, compare a beef steak from a range-fed steer or a wild deer with one from a pen-fed steer. The muscle tissue from the active steer or wild animal is tough and dense; the pen-fed steer's muscle tissue is marbled with fat. Fat marbling makes a steer's muscles tender and juicy; but we have other uses for *our* muscles. This fat marbling explains how we can have a large amount of our muscle replaced with fat as we grow older and yet not gain much weight. The heavier protein tissue is being replaced with lighter fat tissue. Eventually the muscle replacement will stop and then the fat becomes deposited in the adipose tissue under our skin, and we realize we are getting fat.

How does this fat marbling affect our energy expenditure? As we have shown, resting muscle requires about 300 calories of energy a day for a woman and 400 calories for a man. As your muscle tissue is replaced by fat, this energy need will decrease proportionately since fat cells require much less energy than resting muscle cells. Also, as you lose muscle tissue, your ability to be physically active decreases, so you need less energy for muscle motion. As your need for energy decreases, your body will burn less fuel and the excess fuel from your food will be stored as fat. Your greater fat stores will cause you to be even less active. Your decreased activity will lead to greater fat marbling. Soon you are in the midst of a vicious cycle, illustrated on p. 38.

If you are one of the many caught in this vicious cycle, can you do anything about it? Can the cycle be broken and the processes reversed? Several recent studies have shown that you can get out of the cycle by deliberately increasing your physical activity. The increased physical activity will cause your body to replace the fat marbling with muscle tissue. (Women need not be concerned about becoming "muscle bound"; the maximum amount of muscle you can de-

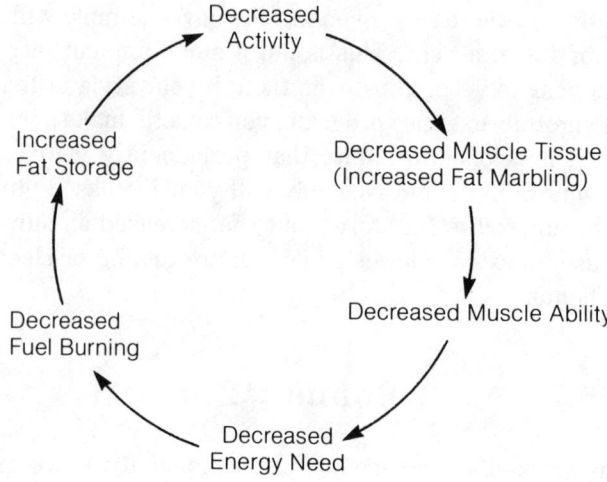

velop is determined by your sex hormones.) When you replace fat marbling with muscle tissue, you bring your muscles back up to your particular capacity.

Energy is required to build and maintain the additional muscle cells that your activity is causing your body to build. Your body will also have to build new mitochondria powerhouses and new fuel-burning enzymes to produce the needed energy for the manufacture and use of the new muscle tissue. The extra energy will require more fuel, so your fat cells will mobilize additional fat to provide the fatty acids for the muscle mitochondria to burn for energy. Your new muscle tissue will enable your body to become more active; you will burn more fuel for the increased muscle motion. The increased muscle motion will cause your body to replace more of the fat marbling with muscle tissue; and soon you will find yourself in a beneficial cycle:

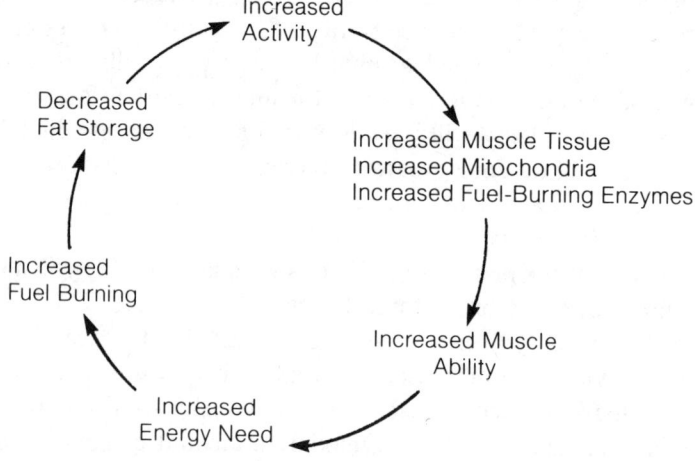

Thus your increased physical activity will make your body capable of sustaining even greater activity. The increased activity will use energy for the muscle motion, but will also use energy to manufacture the new muscle tissue, and to maintain the new muscle tissue while you are resting. This is the double bonus that enables you to burn up calories while you are sleeping.

But this is not all. Your increased physical activity will improve your general health. This is your third bonus.

Bonus #3

During those same years that your decreased physical activity was causing your body to replace muscle tissue with fat, other changes were also taking place. Your heart muscles were becoming weakened because you seldom caused your heart to beat vigorously. Your weakened heart muscle had to beat more often to pump your blood around your body, so your pulse rate went up. Your arteries accumulated fat deposits, so your blood pressure increased. The muscles around your lungs were seldom used to capacity, so they too became weakened, which resulted in less oxygen intake per breath. These changes resulted in a smaller volume of blood, and hence smaller amounts of nutrients and oxygen reaching your individual cells.

Drastic complications result from the deprived cells. Bone cells lose some of their minerals and become brittle and less dense. Nerve cells deteriorate. Heart muscle becomes further weakened and more prone to failure. In addition inactivity leads to tendon and ligament constriction that result in aches, pain, stiffness, and fatigue. In fact it is believed by some that many of the body conditions that are blamed on old age really are a result of a lifetime of inactivity. Inactivity contributes to another kind of vicious cycle:

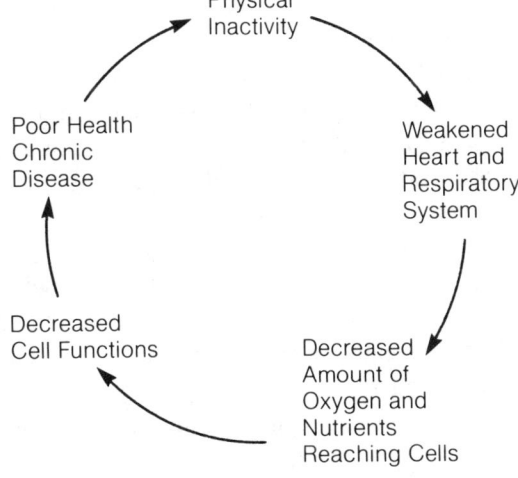

Just as with fat marbling of your muscles, the only way to break out of this vicious cycle is to increase your physical activity—get up and move! Make yourself participate in some physical activity that is regular and active enough to increase your heartbeat and respiration rate. This regular activity, which will strengthen your heart and respiratory muscles, will result in a greater amount of oxygen and nutrients being pumped to your cells. With increased nutrients and oxygen the metabolic functions of your cells will improve. The improved functions will result in better health, which will result in increased physical activity. And you will find yourself in another beneficial cycle:

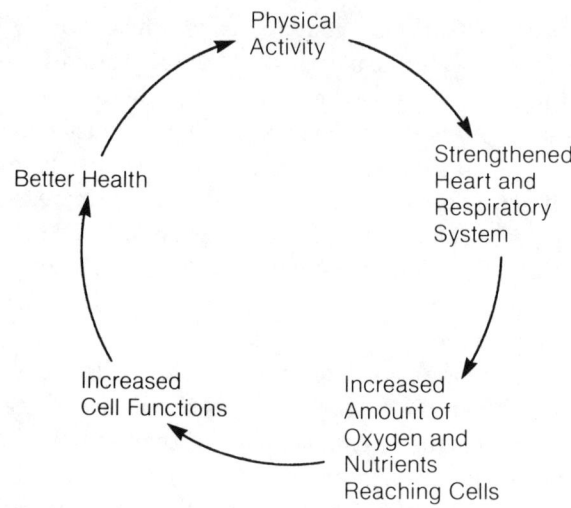

As the flow of blood—with its heightened content of nutrients and oxygen —is increased to your individual cells, several clinical improvements will be noted. Your pulse rate will be lowered because the stronger heart muscles can beat fewer times to send the blood through the body. The increased blood flow will also open up capillaries, thus lowering your blood pressure by decreasing the resistance to flow. The strengthened heart muscle and expanded capillaries will decrease your risks for cardiovascular diseases such as heart attacks and strokes. And your body fat will be reduced because of the increased need for energy to power your more active muscles.

And this is not all. Not only will your physical health improve, but, as most active people will verify, you will feel, look, and work better. Scientists have noted that physical activity also improves one's mental or psychological health. It has been found that physically active persons have less tension. (A walk after a tense day is more relaxing than a drink.) Active persons have increased self-confidence, increased ability to concentrate, and better attitudes and performance at work.

Actually there is a fourth bonus: research has shown that the control of hunger and appetite works quite well in active people and only fails when activity falls below a certain minimum level. Overweight persons, after becoming physically active, have noted a reduced desire to eat excessively. Thus, when overweight persons become active, they are much better able to control their food intake.

Recent research is bringing to light two other bonuses of physical activity: resistance to pain and a euphoric (happy) feeling. It has been found that physical activity results in an increased production of brain peptides known as *endorphins* and *enkelphins*. These brain peptides are believed to be involved in the transmission of pain to the brain, and also involved in mood changes. Hence it is believed that the peptides are responsible for decreased pain sensitivity and for the "runner's high."

Perhaps you resist increasing your levels of activity because the currently popular jogging, handball, tennis, etc., would be too dramatic a change for your budget, time, and personality to fit your style of living. Two things should be remembered: First, *any* increase of physical activity will pay dividends. Second, the dividends increase as the level increases. The important thing is to start now —today, with some sort of program. This one single change in your life can make it possible for you to lose weight, improve your shape, burn unwanted calories while you sleep, diminish your appetite, and improve your sense of self-worth. That's a pretty impressive payoff. Don't resist. Don't postpone. Do it now.

CHAPTER 5

The Devil Made Me Do It

Introduction

Have you ever found yourself putting food into your mouth when you knew you weren't hungry? What made you do it? Once it was fashionable to blame such things on fate, on the gods, or on the devil. Now it is believed that we eat because of signals that reach our brains. As we explained in Chapter 1, your appestat receives signals from sensors in your digestive system, your blood, and perhaps your fat cells. Your appestat then sends signals to your higher brain centers and you decide to eat or to stop eating. However, these signals from your appestat can be overridden by signals from external stimuli. When you respond repeatedly to a given signal, you develop a habit. Then when the signal is present, you respond without even being aware that an external signal, rather than hunger, made you want to eat. Many of these eating habits were developed in childhood and have become a part of your life-style.

Principles of Behavior Modification

There are several steps necessary to overcome habits that lead to overeating. These steps are (1) to become aware of the habits that lead you to overeat; (2) to set goals for yourself; (3) to rearrange your environment so that you can accomplish your goal; (4) to practice each small step that will lead to your goal; (5) to reward yourself for your accomplishments; and (6) to make a commitment to continue your goal for an ever-increasing length of time until this goal becomes part of your life-style.

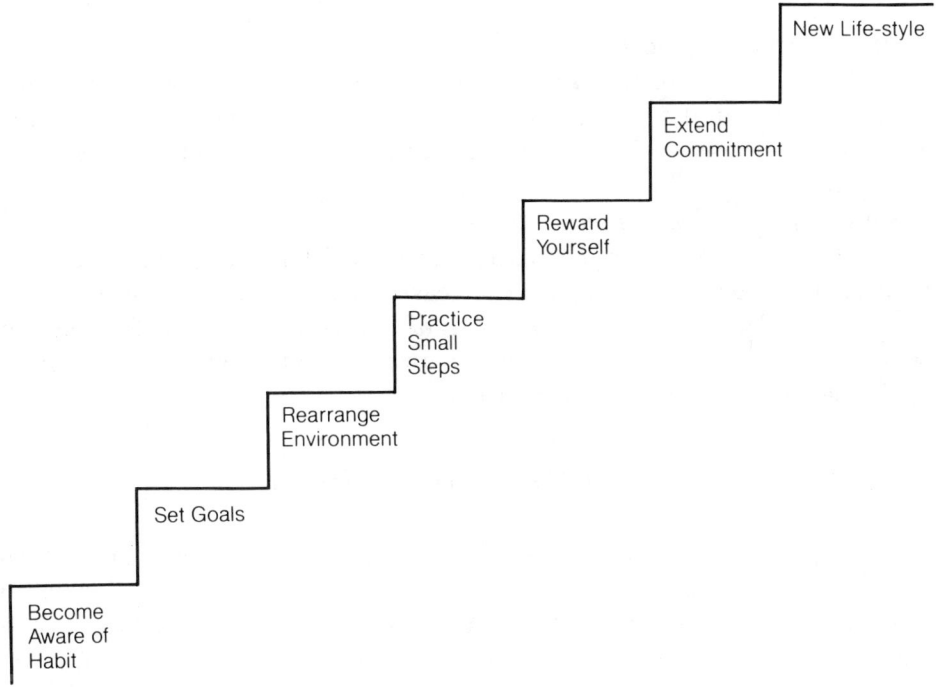

Step 1. *Become aware of habit.*
You can become aware of the habits that lead you to overeat by keeping a very careful record of when, where, and how each time you eat any food. Then you analyze this record to determine what type of stimuli are sending you signals that make you want to eat. You must keep your own record because the stimuli that make you eat may be different from the stimuli that affect others.

Step 2. *Set goals.*
The most important thing about setting goals is that you set them for a short enough time span that you *can* achieve them. You must, at all costs, avoid failure at this point. If a week is too long, set the goal for three days, or one day —but set it so you will succeed.

Step 3. *Rearrange your environment.*

Let your environment work for you rather than against you. But here again, avoid drastic changes. You can live with small changes, such as removing unwanted stimuli from your sight.

Step 4. *Practice small steps.*

After you decide on your goals and rearrange your environment, practice small steps that lead to your goals. Make the steps small enough that you will succeed.

Step 5. *Reward yourself.*

Each time you are successful in accomplishing one step toward your goal for a short period of time, give yourself a nonfood reward. Select enjoyable, appropriate rewards, such as a movie, a magazine, a book, a call to a friend, etc.

Step 6. *Extend your commitment.*

When you find you are successful in accomplishing your goal for a short period of time, commit yourself to an increased time period. Continue increasing the time period until the goal becomes part of your new life-style. Let us consider some of the external stimuli that make you want to eat, and show how you can apply the six principles in managing those stimuli.

Food-Presence Stimuli

The presence of food is probably the strongest of all external stimuli. Who has not found the sight of a newly frosted cake or the smell of freshly baked rolls to be a mouth-watering experience? Even pictures of food, such as in a magazine or on TV, might cause you to want to eat. Somewhere in your past you may have developed the habit of responding to such signals by eating. Let us consider how you might change this habit by following the six principles.

Let us take Norma Taylor for an example. Norma has a habit of eating whenever and wherever food is available. She usually has a plate of cookies on the kitchen counter (for the children when they come home from school). There are dishes of candy and nuts on the coffee table in the living room (in case guests arrive unexpectedly). Chips and dip are usually found near the TV (for something to do when the program is dull). Usually there are pieces of leftover cake or pie at the front of the refrigerator. (Not enough for a meal.) Norma loves to bake.

Norma kept her food record for a week and found she was snacking everywhere and anytime there was food available. She set a goal to eat only at mealtimes for one week. She rearranged her environment by keeping all food out of sight. She continued her baking, but now she put the cookies in a jar on the top shelf of the cabinet. She removed the snack dishes, putting the snacks at the back of the bottom shelf of the refrigerator. The leftover cake and pies were put into the freezer.

As Norma was doing her housework, each time she had a strong desire for a snack, she went for a ten-minute walk around the block. After each walk she put a checkmark on her calendar; for every ten checks she treated herself to a new magazine. For every day that she succeeded in eating only at mealtimes, she deposited fifty cents in her piggy bank to be used for the new dress she would buy when she attained a smaller dress size. After she found that she could succeed for a week, she extended her goal for two weeks, then a month.

PRINCIPLE	PROCEDURE
1. BECOME AWARE OF HABIT.	1. KEEP FOOD RECORD FOR A WEEK; ANALYZE FOOD RECORD.
2. SET A GOAL.	2. DECIDE TO EAT ONLY AT MEALTIMES.
3. REARRANGE ENVIRONMENT.	3. KEEP ALL SNACK FOOD OUT OF SIGHT.
4. PRACTICE.	4. TAKE A 10 MIN WALK OR A 10 MIN ROPE JUMP EACH TIME HAVE URGE TO SNACK.
5. REWARD YOURSELF.	5. CHECKMARKS ON CALENDAR; NEW MAGAZINE FOR 10 CHECKS; NEW DRESS FOR EACH SMALLER DRESS SIZE.
6. EXTEND COMMITMENT.	6. EXTEND FOR 2 WEEKS, A MONTH, 2 MONTHS.

Nonfood Stimuli

Other stimuli, although not as obvious as the presence of food, are just as prevalent. For example, the TV commercial—regardless of what is advertised—is a signal for everyone to head for the kitchen to get a snack before the program resumes. For some people reading is a signal to eat—curl up with a good novel and your favorite cookies. For other people a clothes shopping trip must always be accompanied by a stop at the snack bar.

Let's take the case of Alan Graham. Alan's children are grown and gone, his wife works and is too tired in the evenings to do anything, so there isn't much for Alan to do after he comes home except watch TV. Each time the commercial comes on, Alan uses it for an excuse to fix himself "just another bite to eat." Alan isn't hungry, but eating gives him something to do. Alan has gained twenty-five pounds in the last five years.

Alan kept a food record for a week and found that he was eating good meals with his wife, but he was snacking during every TV program in the evenings and on weekends. He set a goal to avoid snacks while watching TV. He decided that during each commercial he would work on making a belt with his new leather-craft kit. He put the tool kit and leather right next to the TV so he would remember. Each time a commercial came on, he picked up the belt and carved some additional designs. Halfway through the belt he treated himself to a new specialized tool. Soon he had the belt finished; so he extended his commitment to make a belt for each of his children.

PRINCIPLE	PROCEDURE
1. BECOME AWARE OF HABIT.	1. KEEP A FOOD RECORD FOR A WEEK; ANALYZE RECORD.
2. SET A GOAL.	2. DECIDE NOT TO SNACK DURING TV COMMERCIAL.
3. REARRANGE ENVIRONMENT.	3. KEEP LEATHER-CRAFT KIT NEXT TO TV SET.
4. PRACTICE.	4. WORK ON BELT DURING EACH COMMERCIAL.
5. REWARD YOURSELF.	5. A NEW TOOL AFTER COMPLETING HALF A BELT.
6. EXTEND COMMITMENT.	6. MAKE A BELT FOR EACH OF CHILDREN.

Mood Stimuli

Your appestat signals are often overridden by external stimuli, but they are also overridden by signals from your emotions. Over the years you may have found that food helps to relieve problem emotions. So now a certain mood triggers your response to eat. Very early in your life you probably learned that a "goodie" made a hurt feel better. Even though it was the attention of the person giving the "goodie" that helped you, you learned to associate the food with the good feeling. Let us consider problem moods that you might encounter:

Boredom
One of the worst problem moods is boredom. You become bored when you have nothing to do. You also get bored when you are performing a task that is not stimulating to you. You eat to relieve the boredom.

Restlessness
Another problem mood is restlessness, which is often caused by sitting too long. A student studying for finals, a secretary typing a long report, or a bank official examining credit applications get restless. Often, getting up to obtain some food provides the necessary break.

Loneliness

Loneliness is a problem mood. Maybe you are alone this evening, so you eat a box of chocolates in consolation. Maybe you live alone and use food to help your loneliness each evening.

"The Blues"

Another problem emotion is unhappiness—"the blues," "down in the dumps," "depressed." Everything seems to be against you. So you eat the chocolate sundae to "cheer you up." However, you usually are not cheered up; just disgusted at yourself for eating so much. This problem mood is particularly dangerous because it can trap you in a depression-food-depression cycle.

Anger

Sometimes when you are angry, you overeat as if to punish others by stuffing yourself. It seems, at the moment, to be a way to get back at the one causing the anger. Usually all the eating does is to make you angry with yourself.

Worry

Worry is another emotion that might cause you to eat. You usually worry about something that you cannot do anything about at the moment. So you eat in order to have something to do. For example, while you are waiting up for your daughter to get home from a late date, you imagine all kinds of disasters, so you raid the refrigerator to calm yourself.

Let's take the case of Fred Oneto. Fred works for the electric company and spends most of his day at the billing machine. He is bored with his work; he feels he is in a dead-end job. The highlights of his working day are the coffee and doughnuts during the breaks. He also keeps candy in his desk drawer for something to munch on between breaks.

Fred kept a food record at home and at work. He found he was eating regular, balanced meals at home and was too busy in the evenings to be bothered with snacks. However, he found that he was eating almost constantly while at work. He set a goal to avoid all snacks at work for at least a week. He rearranged his environment by giving away the candy in his desk drawer and by agreeing with a coworker to walk at least four blocks during each coffee break. He rewarded himself with fifty cents each time he went for a walk, and with one dollar for each day he succeeded in going without a snack at work. The money was to be used to buy a new tennis racquet so he and his coworker could join the company tennis team. He extended his commitment to continue his walking until he had enough money to buy the racquet and join the tennis team.

PRINCIPLE	PROCEDURE
1. BECOME AWARE OF HABIT.	1. KEEP FOOD RECORD FOR A WEEK; ANALYZE FOOD RECORD.
2. SET A GOAL.	2. DECIDE TO AVOID SNACKS AT WORK.
3. REARRANGE ENVIRONMENT.	3. GIVE AWAY CANDY; TAKE WALKS DURING BREAKS.
4. PRACTICE.	4. WALK WITH COWORKER EACH DAY DURING BREAKS.
5. REWARD YOURSELF.	5. BANK 50¢ FOR EACH WALK ; $ 1 FOR EACH SUCCESSFUL DAY.
6. EXTEND COMMITMENT.	6. CONTINUE WALKS UNTIL ENOUGH MONEY FOR NEW TENNIS RACQUET; JOIN COMPANY TENNIS TEAM.

Now let's consider Lois Miller, a twenty-nine-year-old divorcée who lives alone. Lois is one of the best teachers at Evergreen Elementary. Her students are doing outstanding work; but she has a stack of papers to grade each night. Lois usually rests for an hour or so after getting home from work; then she prepares her dinner. After the kitchen cleanup Lois settles down for an evening of paper-grading. Lois kept a food record for a week and found that all of her snacking and most of her food consumption was after 8:00 P.M. and on weekends. Lois set a goal to eat no food at night after dinner for two weeks. To rearrange her environment Lois took her papers to the public library and graded them there. She also joined a Friday-night square-dance group and a weekend hiking club. For each day that she ate no food after dinner, she rewarded herself with one dollar. She extended her commitment to continue grading her papers at the library and to continue attending the square-dance and hiking club activities until she had enough money from her rewards for a new pair of hiking boots and a square-dance outfit.

PRINCIPLE	PROCEDURE
1. BECOME AWARE OF HABIT.	1. KEEP FOOD RECORD FOR A WEEK; ANALYZE FOOD RECORD.
2. SET A GOAL.	2. DECIDE TO EAT NO FOOD AFTER DINNER FOR 2 WEEKS.
3. REARRANGE ENVIRONMENT.	3. GO TO LIBRARY TO GRADE PAPERS; GET INVOLVED IN WEEKEND ACTIVITIES.
4. PRACTICE.	4. GRADE PAPERS AT LIBRARY; ATTEND WEEKEND ACTIVITIES.
5. REWARD YOURSELF.	5. $ 1 FOR EACH DAY WITH NO FOOD AFTER DINNER.
6. EXTEND COMMITMENT.	6. CONTINUE TO GRADE PAPERS IN LIBRARY AND TO ATTEND WEEKEND ACTIVITIES UNTIL REWARD MONEY WILL BUY NEW HIKING BOOTS AND DANCE OUTFIT.

Responding to environmental stimuli (to eat food) over a period of time creates self-defeating habits. Signals that lead to overeating can be diminished by gradually replacing the eating habits with other habits. As you develop new habits, you will be changing your way of living. Gradually, as you change your life-style, you will become a slim person who will remain slim for life.

CHAPTER 6

Fad Diets—Solutions or Illusions?

Introduction

Everyone wants a quick, easy way to lose fat. Books or gimmicks that promise quick, effortless ways to reduce are bought in great numbers. "Calories don't count," "diet revolution," "drink all you want," "lose forty pounds in two weeks," are some of the promises. Fad diets do result in weight loss; but when the diet is over, the weight usually is regained in a remarkably short time. The dieter then finds another diet book that makes even more lavish promises than the last book. This diet is tried, weight is lost, the diet is given up, and the weight is regained. Most dieters find that over the long run they maintain a fairly stable weight regardless of the number of diets tried.

The popular, quick weight-loss diets have one characteristic in common—they are unbalanced nutritionally. Nearly all are deficient in vitamins and minerals—some more than others. As you learned in previous chapters, balance is required by the body in order to carry on its functions. Let us consider specific types of fad diets and how their particular imbalance affects the body.

Fasting

Fasting, or very low-calorie diets, has been promoted as the quickest way to lose weight. These diets are just voluntary starvation and the body goes into a tailspin trying to preserve life during starvation. Total fasting or very low-calorie diets should be used only under very close medical supervision. Let us consider some of the events that take place during starvation.

The average person requires about 150 grams of glucose per day to provide fuel for the brain and other tissues that can use only glucose. The blood normally contains about a 20-gram reserve and liver glycogen another 80 to 90 grams. (Muscle glycogen can be used only by the muscle.) So in less than one day of starvation the body runs out of its glucose reserve for the brain. At this point the body begins to break down its own muscle tissue to obtain amino acids to be converted to glucose. The muscle tissue is lost not only from the arms and legs, but also from the heart, liver, kidneys, and skin. The body also breaks down stored fat and uses the fatty acids for energy for tissues that do not require glucose. However, in starvation there is not enough glucose present to burn the fatty acids completely; instead ketone bodies are formed. The ketones enter the blood and the person goes into a state of ketosis, with symptoms such as fatigue, nausea, irritability, and dizziness. If the fast is continued for a long enough period of time, the brain adapts to utilizing ketones for energy in an effort to spare the vital protein tissues; however, the brain still requires 50 percent of its energy from glucose. The basal metabolic rate slows down, as much as 50 percent, in an effort to conserve the available fuel. Muscle activity is also drastically curtailed. A result of these conserving measures is that much less fat is burned than would be expected from the calorie deficit. After the fast is ended, the weight lost is rapidly regained. However, because of the reduced basal metabolism and decreased activity, much of the lost protein is replaced with fat. So the person ends up with the same weight but a greater percent fat than before the fast.

Protein-Sparing Modified Fast

To prevent the protein loss that accompanied total fasting, the protein-sparing modified fast was instituted. This fast was designed for clinical use, where it appears to have some value. However, it entered the popular press in diets such as "The Last Chance Diet," in which fasting was to be accompanied by liquid protein. Apparently the diet may be just that—your last chance—to do anything. Most of the liquid protein mixes were made from collagen (a protein from beef hides). Collagen is about the most biologically inadequate protein there is. Deaths were reported of people on this diet, even when under medical supervision. A recent study by the University of Rochester Medical Center has found that the liquid-protein diets are directly associated with life-threatening heart irregularities. The American Medical Association recommends that the liquid-protein diet be restricted to the grossly obese and used under a doctor's supervision, with vitamin and mineral supplements.

Low-Carbohydrate Diets

The most popular of the current diets are the low-carbohydrate diets. Carbohydrate has become the whipping boy, since carbohydrates are found in such goodies as candy, cookies, and cake. Controlled studies have shown that there is a greater weight loss while on a low-carbohydrate diet than on a balanced diet of the same number of calories. However it has also been shown that the additional weight loss is due to a loss of body water, rather than body fat. Water is necessary for the binding of glycogen, the storage form of carbohydrates. On a low-carbohydrate diet the liver glycogen is rapidly depleted, along with its bound water. Body proteins also require water for binding; when these proteins are converted to glucose, that water is also lost. In addition low-carbohydrate diets are accompanied by an excessive loss of body fluids. When a person goes "off the diet," the water is rapidly replaced, so the lost weight is quickly regained.

The low-carbohydrate diets are either high protein or high fat or both. Both fats and protein require glucose for complete burning to provide energy. When there is insufficient glucose, the incomplete burning of fatty acids or amino acids forms ketone bodies, which enter the bloodstream and cause ketosis. In addition to the symptoms suffered by adults, ketone bodies are known to cause brain damage to a developing fetus. Low-carbohydrate diets should be strictly avoided by women who are pregnant—or who might be pregnant, since the greatest damage takes place in the first trimester, when pregnancy is often unrecognized.

High-Protein Diets

The most popular of the low-carbohydrate diets are the high-protein diets. These diets often consist of a low-carbohydrate food diet, accompanied by expensive protein powder supplements. (These diets are often advocated by persons or organizations who are selling the protein powders.)

In addition to the problems caused by the low carbohydrates the high-protein diets overload the kidneys. The body can use only a certain amount of protein to provide amino acids to build the body's own proteins; any excess must be converted to fat or burned for energy. In both the conversion to fat and the burning for energy there is a nitrogen waste product that must be excreted by the kidneys. Kidney damage is one of the complications of prolonged high-protein diets. Anyone with kidney disease is warned to avoid high-protein diets. These diets also result in an accumulation of another nitrogen waste product, called *uric acid,* which may cause gout in susceptible persons. Recent research has shown that high-protein diets cause a loss of bone calcium and may result in osteoporosis. Another problem with the high-protein, low-carbohydrate diets is that they usually are low in dietary fiber. Digestive disorders will be the least of the complications of these diets.

High-Fat Diets

The early low-carbohydrate diets were also high-fat diets. These diets advocated high fat as a way to get rid of storage fat. (The logic eludes us.) In addition to the complications associated with low-carbohydrate diets, such as ketosis, excessive fluid loss, and lack of fiber, high fat diets have recently been found to be a strong risk factor in coronary heart disease. This danger is now so widely accepted that high-fat diets are no longer advocated.

Vegetarian Diets

The vegetarian diets advocate high carbohydrate, low protein, and low fat. These diets can be an excellent way to lose weight if care is taken to obtain complementary protein foods, and to obtain supplements of vitamin B_{12} and iron. However, most vegetarian diets designed for weight loss advocate lots and lots of salad greens plus rice. It is hardly possible for most persons to eat enough salad greens to obtain sufficient protein; and rice by itself is an incomplete protein. A mild protein deficiency will result in decreased resistance to infection because there are insufficient amino acids to build the antibodies and white blood cells to fight infection. Another complication of protein deficiency is poor wound healing caused also by insufficient amounts of the needed amino acids.

High-Fiber Diet

Another type of diet being advocated is the high-fiber diet, which advocates adding bran to the ordinary diet. If the diet is otherwise balanced, addition of fiber may be an aid to weight reduction. However adding fiber (particularly wood fiber) to an unbalanced diet may cause more harm than good—possibly causing digestive problems such as ulcers and diverticulitis. Also bran fiber can "bind" with minerals in the intestine and prevent their absorption.

Comparison of Diets

Much research has been done on diets of all kinds; the results have not been encouraging. Fad diets cause a weight loss, but since they do not cause a person to change his or her life-style in any way, the weight is promptly regained when the diet is ended. Very low-calorie and low-carbohydrate diets, in addition to the clinical problems, are deceptive in that the person thinks he or she is losing fat, when the loss is mostly body water.

In 1967, an authoritative study was performed by Drs. Yang and Van Itallie in New York. Very obese males were placed on a regime that consisted of three ten-day periods during which the subjects were (1) starved, (2) received an 800-calorie low-carbohydrate diet, or (3) received an 800-calorie balanced diet. The subjects were placed on a 1200-calorie balanced diet in the interval between each of the ten-day periods. The experiment began and ended with two further 1200-calorie periods. The results of the study are given in Table 7 and in Figure 11. These results have been verified by a more recent study.

TABLE 7 COMPARISON OF DIETS

TYPE OF DIET	EXPERIMENTAL PERIOD				POSTEXPERIMENTAL PERIOD
	WEIGHT LOSS	WATER LOSS	FAT LOSS	PROTEIN LOSS	WEIGHT CHANGE
STARVATION	−751 G/D	−458 G/D	−243 G/D	−50.4 G/D	145 G/D
LOW-CARBOHYDRATE	−467 G/D	−284 G/D	−165 G/D	−17.9 G/D	145 G/D
BALANCED	−278 G/D	− 53 G/D	−165 G/D	−9.5 G/D	−165 G/D

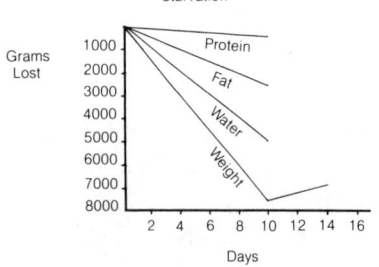 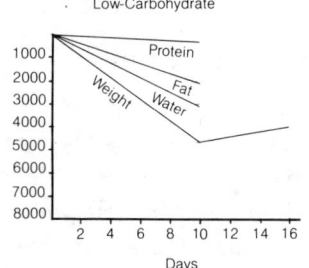 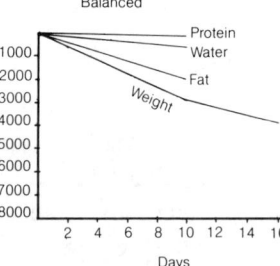

Fig. 11   Comparison of Diets

THE BIO-PLAN FOR LIFELONG WEIGHT CONTROL

This study showed that starvation and low-carbohydrate diets definitely result in a greater weight loss than does a balanced diet. However, most of the weight-loss difference was due to water loss. Starvation resulted in the greatest loss of fat, but also in a much greater loss of lean body tissue (protein) than either a low-carbohydrate or balanced diet. A very interesting point to note was that after the starvation and low-carbohydrate diets were discontinued, weight was regained at a rate of 145 grams per day. But after the balanced diet was discontinued, weight continued to be lost at a rate of 165 grams per day. Most of the immediate postexperimental weight gain of the men after the starvation and the low-carbohydrate diets was due to a replacement of body water. After the balanced diet there was not that much water to replace and the men could continue to lose fat on a 1200-calorie diet.

Drugs

Some persons find that they can't lose weight fast enough on a fad diet, so they resort to drugs. The drugs used most commonly are laxatives, diuretics, appetite suppressants, and hormones. Laxatives are used simply to make the food move through the intestinal tract too fast to be absorbed. The laxatives also prevent essential vitamins and minerals from being absorbed. Diuretics are used to force the body to remove more water, and hence result in a weight loss. Diuretics have some value for a person who is retaining too much water; although a reduction in salt intake will accomplish the same result, without the mineral loss caused by diuretics. For a normal person diuretics may result in dehydration.

Some of the appetite suppressants are the amphetamines, such as Dexedrine, and fenfluramines, such as pondimin, which are central nervous system stimulants. The appetite suppression seems to result from the person being "all wired up" and too "high" to want to eat. The possibilities for emotional, and perhaps physical, addiction are great. Another appetite suppressant, phenyl-propanolamine (PPA), which can be obtained without a prescription, is supposed to act by sending "full" signals to the appestat. PPA appears not to have the stimulant action of the other appetite suppressants. However, some studies indicate that PPA elevates blood pressure and this could be dangerous in a person with hypertension. Also serious side effects have been noted when PPA is combined with other medications. But the main drawback to drugs is that unless the person changes his life-style, he is committed to a lifelong dependency on that drug to help maintain his desired weight.

Another type of appetite suppressant is the bulk-forming agents. These are mainly methylcellulose, a wood product which expands by absorbing water from the stomach, giving the feeling of fullness. The same effect can be obtained at a much lower cost, from the fiber found in fruits, vegetables, and whole grains.

Thyroid extracts are sometimes given with the aim of increasing the person's basal metabolism and hence energy output. The drug is helpful if the person does suffer from an underactive thyroid. However, for normal, healthy persons the drug can throw the entire hormone system of the body out of balance. Some side effects that have been noted are the risks of depleting lean body mass and of irritating the heart muscle.

The use of the human chorionic gonadotropin (HCG) hormone was introduced in 1961. It was supposed to cause a pregnancylike condition in which body fat is mobilized rapidly for the needs of a growing fetus. In nonpregnant persons, men or women, it is said that the hormone is not activated unless the person is restricted to a 500-calorie diet. This weight-loss scheme has been shown to be an expensive, ineffective ripoff. The weight loss on a 500-calorie diet with HCG has been shown to be no different from that which results from a balanced 500-calorie diet without HCG. Side effects of the drug include headache, restlessness, depression; long-term effects are not known but could be potentially dangerous.

Bypass Surgery

For very obese persons neither diet nor drugs are effective. In these cases two types of surgery have been tried. Although the surgical remedies cannot be classed as fad diets, they are still largely in the experimental stage and should be resorted to only after careful consideration.

The first type of weight-control surgery is the intestinal bypass in which part of a person's small intestine is tied off. The shorter intestine results in less food being absorbed and much more being wasted. Patients, after intestinal bypass surgery, do lose some weight, but do not stabilize at normal levels. Complications following this type of surgery include electrolyte and essential mineral loss, liver disease, bone demineralization, and kidney stones. It is recommended that the procedure be limited to those who have been over 200 percent of their ideal weight for more than a year. It is stressed that because of the uncertainty of long-term liver disease and prolonged electrolyte loss, the bypass should be performed only in well-staffed hospitals where adequate follow-up is available.

The second type of surgery, known as the gastric bypass, consists of stapling off a portion of the stomach. The smaller stomach can hold only a limited amount of food, so the surgery is an effective food-intake control. However, gastric bypass surgery is still in the experimental stage and is potentially hazardous. The recommendations are the same as for the intestinal bypass.

Fad diets and drugs contribute to the yo-yo effect that many dieting Americans undergo. The repeated failures just convince people that *they* are failures and cannot lose weight. And in many instances the accompanying nutritional imbalance damages the body temporarily, if not permanently. How, then, can you safely and permanently lose weight? Only by applying the principles in the preceding chapters to a permanent, comfortable modification of your life-style.

CHAPTER 7

The Only Way

Now that you have come this far in this book, you know what makes people fat and what is necessary to get rid of the fat. You know that for permanent weight control, crash diets do not work, drugs do not work, and starvation does not work. You understand that the only thing that does work is for you to change your life-style in such a way that you trade those behaviors that lead to fat storage for behaviors that lead to fat utilization.

"That's all very fine," you say, "but not for me. I could never do all those things. I'll never be a slim person." To you becoming a slim person is like trying to climb to the top of a steep mountain. "I never was good at mountain climbing," you say.

But wait a minute! No one said you had to climb up the face of the cliff. Some people can climb steep cliffs. But for most of us there is a much easier way to get to the top of the mountain. We can follow a trail that gradually switchbacks up the side of the mountain and eventually reaches the top. You can follow this trail and make it to the top because the trail is not extremely steep at any point. The winding trail is longer, but you probably will get to the top of the mountain faster than those people who are trying to climb the face of the cliff. They are probably slipping back ten steps for every five steps forward. And most

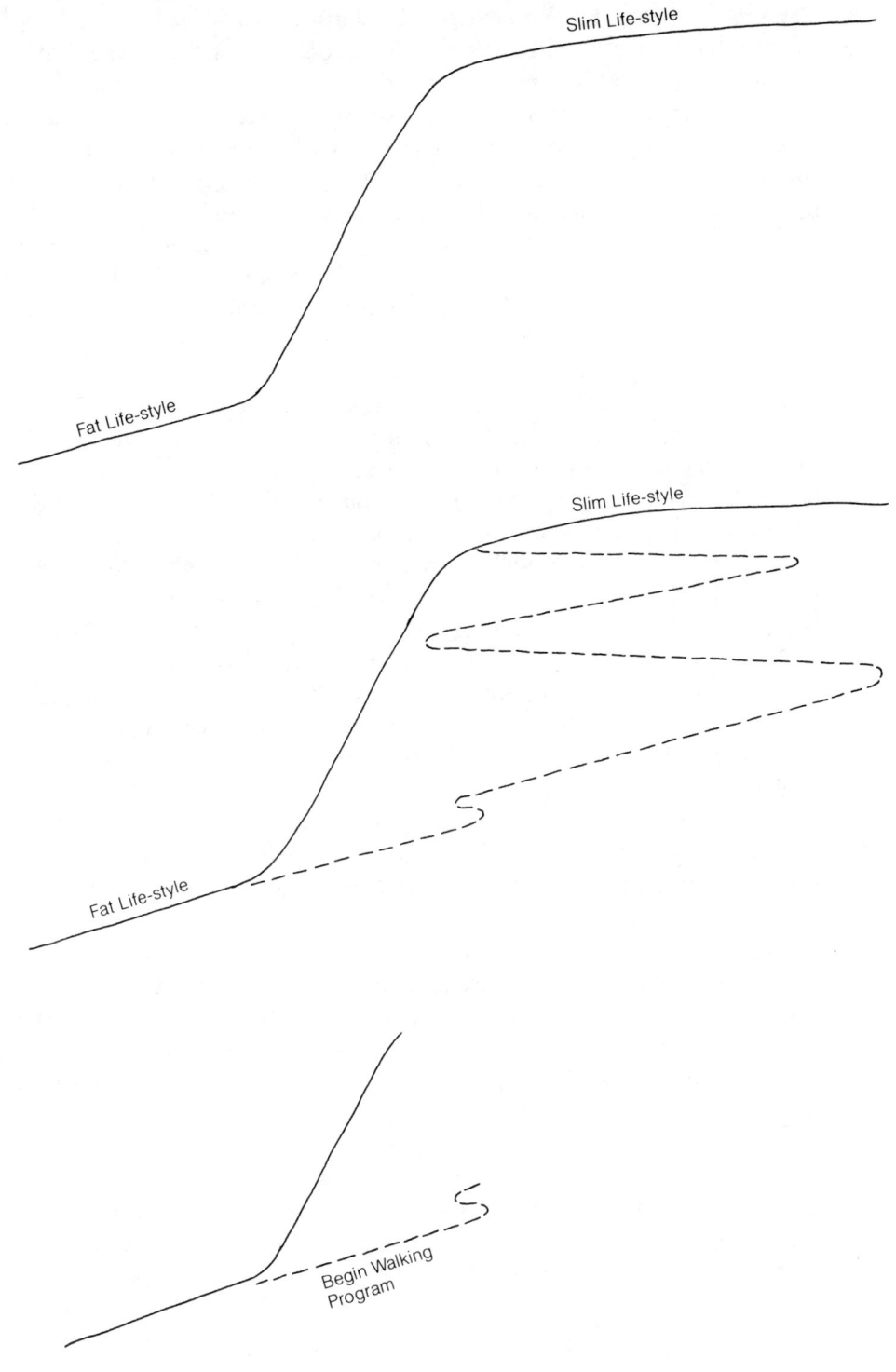

Slim Life-style

Fat Life-style

Slim Life-style

Fat Life-style

Begin Walking
Program

of them will probably give up after the third slip backward.

The first step in becoming a slim person is the same as the first step in climbing a mountain. You must *believe* that you can. Belief is a principle of great power. Once you have an idea or belief about yourself, it becomes "true" as far as you personally are concerned. You will act like the sort of person that you conceive yourself to be. To get to the top of a mountain you must first really want to do so. Then you think about it, daydream about it, and picture yourself at the top. It is the same with becoming a slim person. Picture in your mind the person you want to become. Daydream: How does a slim person walk? How does a slim person act? Imagine yourself going through the day acting as if you were a slim person. By consistently acting "as if" something is true, in time you can make it become true.

The earlier chapters in this book have described the trail to the top of the mountain. You know the trail is there and you know that other people have followed the trail to the top. Maybe it seems overwhelming to you to try to climb to the top of the mountain, but at least you can go to the first turn in the trail. Almost anyone can begin a walking program.

A walking program will do wonders for you. It makes your heart start pumping harder. And when more oxygen and nutrients reach your cells, the cells begin to function better. Soon you feel good. Not just physically. Your sense of self-worth increases. "I have to be of some value; I've been able to stick to a walking program for three weeks now." It's like realizing that you have been able to make it up to the first turn in the trail. "Hey, I've been able to make it this far; I believe I can go a bit farther." So you try it to the next turn in the trail.

Walking feels so good that now you decide you will walk, or run, or jog, or bicycle at your training level. That's really getting the blood where you want it to go. You have reached the first switchback on the trail up your mountain, and the view makes you really want to go on.

Now you concentrate on the nutrients that you are sending to your cells. You have to have the right nutrients to provide the necessary energy and building materials for your cells. So now you learn to plan and eat nutritionally balanced meals. This takes you to the next switchback and the view is breathtaking! You feel so good that you have been able to come this far. (And your body feels so good that it is getting the proper nutrients.)

You are almost to the top of the mountain, and now you know that you can make it the rest of the way. Perhaps you are still having a problem with extra-fuel snacks and eating when you are not hungry. Now is the time to control the external stimuli that override the hunger signals from your appestat. You determine which external stimuli are your problems and set about rearranging your environment such that you can control those signals. And you find that you have

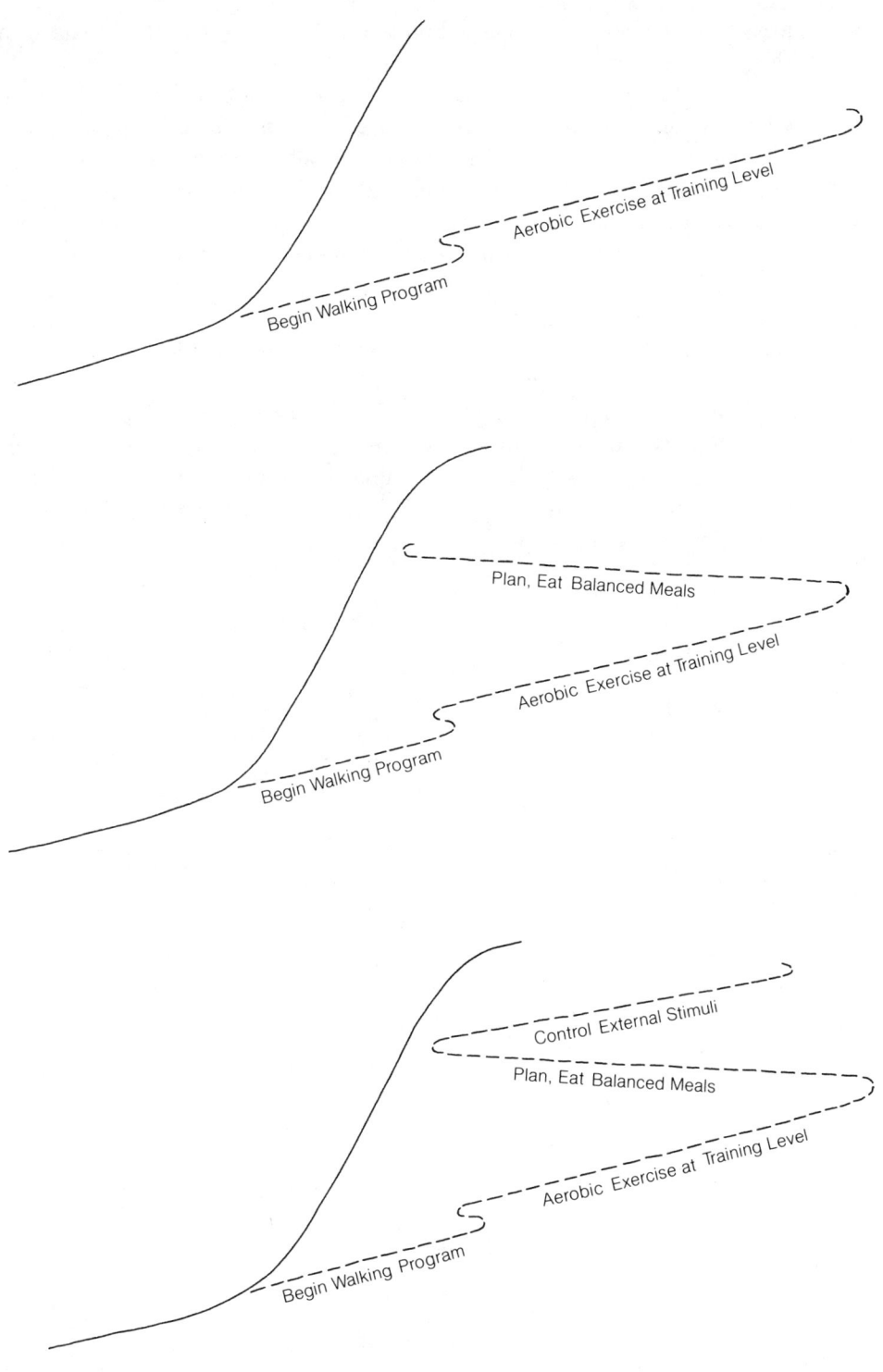

Begin Walking Program

Aerobic Exercise at Training Level

Plan, Eat Balanced Meals

Begin Walking Program

Aerobic Exercise at Training Level

Control External Stimuli

Plan, Eat Balanced Meals

Aerobic Exercise at Training Level

Begin Walking Program

arrived at the next switchback. You realize it's not going to be so hard to reach the top now.

You feel very confident and successful. You are the one in control—not your environment. Except when you are depressed. Something comes up in your life that plunges you into "the depths." Then nothing matters—and you find yourself slipping back into your old eating habits. What can you do? Well, when you are in the midst of "the blues," you probably can't do much of anything— you don't care enough. But prevention is much better than cure. You know that there will be times in your life when you will be "depressed," so you plan ahead. You develop a strategy that you will follow when you become "depressed"; something you will *do*, rather than eat. Then, when the occasion arises, you apply your strategy. Success! After a few successes in following your strategies, you are well along the trail. Now you know that you are going to make it to the top! At last you are at the top of the mountain. When people begin complimenting you on your new look, you realize you have become a slim person. And hey, you *like* this life-style! This is really living! All you have to do now is to maintain the life-style you have adopted.

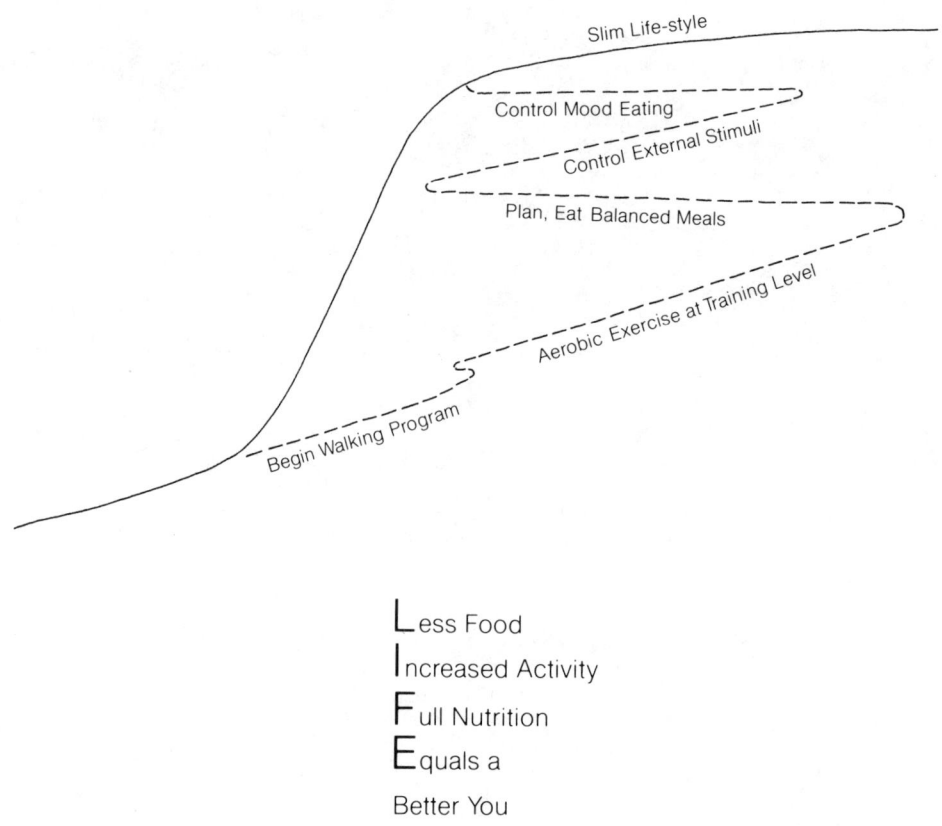

Less Food
Increased Activity
Full Nutrition
Equals a
Better You

This is the trail to the top of the mountain, the pathway to becoming a slim person. It sounds so simple, but you are still hesitant; the description of the path is too general. You want and need more detail to make daily progress. For you all the necessary maps and road signs are in the next section of the book. *Bon voyage!*

PART II.

Planning Your Own Weight-Control Program

Introduction

The object of this portion of our book is to help you develop your own weight-control program. This program will be divided into two parts: The first helps you achieve your optimal weight, and the second allows you to maintain that weight happily, comfortably, and naturally for the rest of your life.

As you develop your weight-control program, you will complete several assignments that will help you practice the principles of weight control. These are listed on the following pages.

Week	Assignment	
1	1	Select a support group of friends; decide on rewards for successful completion of assignments.
1	2	Keep a "food and eating habits" record for one week before beginning your weight-reducing diet.
1	3	Start a "weight and measurement" record.
1	4	Begin a walking program.
3	5	Plan your meals for a week, using one of the basic exchange diets. Then continue until you reach your desired body weight.
5	6	Begin an aerobic exercise program.
5	7	Begin a toning exercise program. (Simultaneous with aerobic exercise.)
5	8	Pay the price for extra-fuel foods with increased physical activity.
8	9	Analyze your "food and behavior" records.
8	10	Practice techniques to control external stimuli.
8	11	Practice techniques to control the amount of your food intake.
8	12	Plan and practice substitutes for mood eating.
11	13	Begin your own exercise program.
14	14	Plan and follow meals according to maintenance exchange diets.

These assignments will require a certain amount of record-keeping. Table 8 is both a chronological arrangement of the assignments and a records form. As you progress in the program, place a checkmark ($\checkmark$) underneath the appropriate X as you complete each week's assignment(s). Place this record in a prominent place in your home, like on the refrigerator.

TABLE 8 ASSIGNMENT SCHEDULE AND RECORD

ASSIGNMENT NUMBER	1	2	3	4	5	6	7	8	9	10	11	12	13	14	15	16	17	18	19	20	21	22	23	24	25	26	27	28	29	30
#1 SUPPORT AND REWARDS																														
#2 FOOD RECORD																														
#3 WEIGHT RECORD																														
#4 WALKING PROGRAM																														
#5 MEAL PLANNING																														
#6 AEROBIC EXERCISE																														
#7 TONING EXERCISES																														
#8 EXTRA-FUEL FOODS																														
#9 FOOD RECORD ANALYSIS																														
#10 EXTERNAL STIMULI																														
#11 FOOD AMOUNTS																														
#12 MOOD EATING																														
#13 YOUR OWN EXERCISE																														
#14 MAINTENANCE MEALS																														

NOTE: Shade in each weekly square over the X as you complete the assignment. ($\rightarrow$) signifies "continue as long as needed."

CHAPTER 8

Getting Off to a Good Start

Making changes in behavior, particularly in physical activity, is difficult at first. You will probably be more successful if you can join with one or more other persons on the program. Select friends, your spouse, coworkers, your children —any persons who are in about the same physical condition as you are, and with whom you can get together for physical activities at least four times each week.

An alternative to having partners is to enroll in a weight-control class at your local high school or community college. In such a class you will find other persons with the same goals who will provide support for you.

For some people achieving a goal is sufficient reward in itself. However, most of us work better for goals if there are tangible rewards along the way. As you progress in your weight-control program, we are asking you to reward yourself for each small achievement. The rewards can be anything that matters to you (except food). Some examples of rewards are going to a movie, taking time to read a special novel, doing needlework, playing golf, calling a friend, and writing personal letters.

ASSIGNMENT #1. *Support and Rewards*
Select one or more persons to be in your support group. List their names

and addresses on Worksheet #1. Also list some possible rewards that you will give yourself for your achievements. A sample worksheet is given on p. 70. Blank worksheets are found in Appendix C.

Record-Keeping

During the course of this program, you will find it helpful to keep many records. Most of the records will show you the progress you are making. To establish a baseline description of your food-eating habits, you need to record your present eating habits. Later you will analyze this record to find out where your eating habit problems lie.

ASSIGNMENT #2. *Food and Behavior Record*
On the record form, Worksheet #2, record every morsel of food that you take into your mouth. Also list the date, time, place, physical position, associated activity, and with whom you were eating. In addition record your mood and degree of hunger at the time you ate the food. (Your record will be more accurate if you place the worksheet in your kitchen or dining room where you can't miss it.) Keep the record for one week at the beginning of your program, and then keep it for one week before you start Assignments #9, #10, #11, #12. A sample record is shown on p. 72, and blank record forms are given in Appendix C.

You will also want to know the progress you are making in losing weight and fat. So at this time you should record your initial body weight and measurements and also make a photographic measurement of your appearance.

WEIGHT-CONTROL CLASS AT_____

STARTING DATE_____TIME_____

OR/AND

FRIENDS—THE PERSONS IN THIS GROUP WILL BE:

NAME	ADDRESS
Lois	2237 Hillview
Jean	1705 Edgemont

REWARDS—THINGS I LIKE TO DO:

Go to the movies, theater, concerts

Play golf

Go clothes-shopping

Read magazines

Write letters

REWARDS—THINGS I WOULD LIKE TO HAVE (NONFOOD):

Books
_____

Magazines
_____

New clothes
_____

Records + tapes
_____

_____

WORKSHEET #2. FOOD AND BEHAVIOR RECORD

NAME _____ DATES _____

Date Times	Place	Physical Position	With Whom?	Assoc. Activity	Mood	Hunger	Food and Amount
5/10 8 A.M.	dining room	sitting	alone	reading paper	happy	5	8oz coffee, 1 tsp sugar, 2 tsp cream, 2 slices toast, 2 tsp margarine
10 A.M.	utility room	sitting	alone	ironing	tired	3	8oz coffee, 1 tsp sug, 2 tsp cream, 1 bun
11:30 A.M.	kitchen	sitting	daughter	talking	tired	3	TV Dinner, ½ tomato juice
2 P.M.	kitchen	standing	daughter	cleaning	tired	2	4 chocolate chip cookies
4:30 P.M.	kitchen	standing	children	preparing dinner	tired	4	1 bite spaghetti, 2 Tsp. frosting, 2 choc. chip cookies
5:30 p.m.	dining room	sitting	family	talking	tired	3	1 serving spaghetti & meat balls, ½ c. green beans, 1 roll, 1 square choc. cake & frosting, 1 c. coffee, 1 tsp sugar, 2 tsp cream
8 P.M.	living room	sitting	husband	watching TV	bored	1	2 squares choc. cake & frosting, 1 c. coffee, 1 tsp sugar, 2 tsp cream
10:30 PM	living room	sitting	husband	watching TV	tired	1	12 oz. Coke, 2 doughnuts
5/11 8:30 A.M.	dining room	sitting	alone	reading paper	content	5	½ c. cereal, 1 orange, 1 c. coffee, 1 tsp sugar, 2 tsp cream
8:50 AM	kitchen	standing	alone	doing dishes	bored	1	2 choc. chip cookies
10:30 AM	living room	standing	alone	dusting	tired	2	handful nuts, 2 candies
11:30 AM	dining room	sitting	daughter	talking	tired	3	1 bowl cr. of chicken soup, 4 crackers, 1 c. coffee, 1 tsp sugar, 2 tsp cream
12:30 P.M.	kitchen	standing	alone	cleaning	tired	2	4 crackers, 2 tsp butter
4 P.M.	Department store	sitting	alone	none	tired	4	12 oz Coke, 2 oz Burger w. bun, 4 oz french fries, 1 dish ice cream
6:30 PM	dining room	sitting	family	talking	unhappy	2	½ c. cole slaw, 1 c. coffee & sug. occ.
8:30 PM	living room	sitting	husband	watching TV	restless	1	2 squares choc. cake w frosting.

9 P.M.	living room	sitting	husband	watching TV	restless	1	10 potato chips, 2 tb sour cr. dip
10 P.M.	bedroom	lying down	alone	reading	tired	1	25 M&M's
5/12 8:30 A.M.	kitchen	sitting	alone	reading paper	happy	5	2 slices toast, 2 tsp butter, 2 tsp jelly, 1c coffee 1 tsp sugar 2 tsp cream
10 AM	grocery store	standing	alone	shopping	hurried	3	2 buns
11:30 am	dining room	sitting	daughter	talking	tired	3	1 cheese sandwich 1c. coffee w. sugar & cr.
4 P.M.	School snack-bar	sitting	son	talking	tired	3	1 frankfurter w. roll, 17 oz Coke
6:30 PM	dining room	sitting	family	talking	tired	2	1 4oz steak, 1 potato w. gravy, 1/2 c. peas, 1 slice bread, 1 pc apple pie, 1 coffee w sugar & cream

NOTE: RATE HUNGER ON A SCALE 0 TO 5, WITH 5 BEING THE MOST HUNGRY.

ASSIGNMENT #3. *Weight and Measurement Record*

On Worksheet #3, record your present body weight and measurements. Continue recording your weight and measurements every week for twenty weeks; after that, record every two weeks for a year. A sample record is given on p. 75 and blank forms are found in Appendix C. Also place a full-length snapshot of yourself in the upper left-hand corner of the flyleaf of this book. Add another snapshot every six months.

You might also want to determine your "ideal" weight. The height/weight table in Appendix B can be used as an approximate guideline. For a more accurate method use the chart and procedure given on p. 172 in Appendix B.

On your weight-loss program you can expect to lose weight—but not at a steady pace. You will probably have a rapid weight loss at the beginning of your restricted diet; this is due to the loss of body water. This water is lost when your salt or carbohydrate intake is decreased. You may have ups and downs in weight loss; this is usually caused by variations in your salt intake and for women by salt retention during the premenstrual period.

As time goes on, you may see a plateau where you will not have any weight loss. These plateaus are caused by several factors. One, as you "burn up" fat in your cells, water is produced; it takes time for this water to reach your bloodstream and be eliminated. Another, if you are exercising regularly while you are losing fat, you will be replacing fat tissue with protein tissue. Since protein is more dense (heavier) than fat, you might even gain a little weight for a while. A third factor causing plateaus is that when you lose weight, you require less energy to carry out a given activity. So as you lose weight, you have to increase your activity level to maintain the same energy usage.

Your measurement decreases will more accurately reflect your loss of fat than will your body weight. (If you can fit into smaller-size clothes, you know you have lost fat even if your scales do not show it.)

If you find that your weight remains on a plateau for a few weeks, do not be concerned; just continue to follow the program. If the weight plateau lasts for several weeks, first cut down on your salt intake, then increase your physical activity.

As you approach your ideal weight, you will find further weight loss more and more difficult to attain. At this point switch to a maintenance diet and do not try to lose any more weight. (Being too thin is as great a health hazard as being too fat.) From now on just maintain your weight at the new level.

IDEAL WEIGHT
WEIGHT RESPONSE

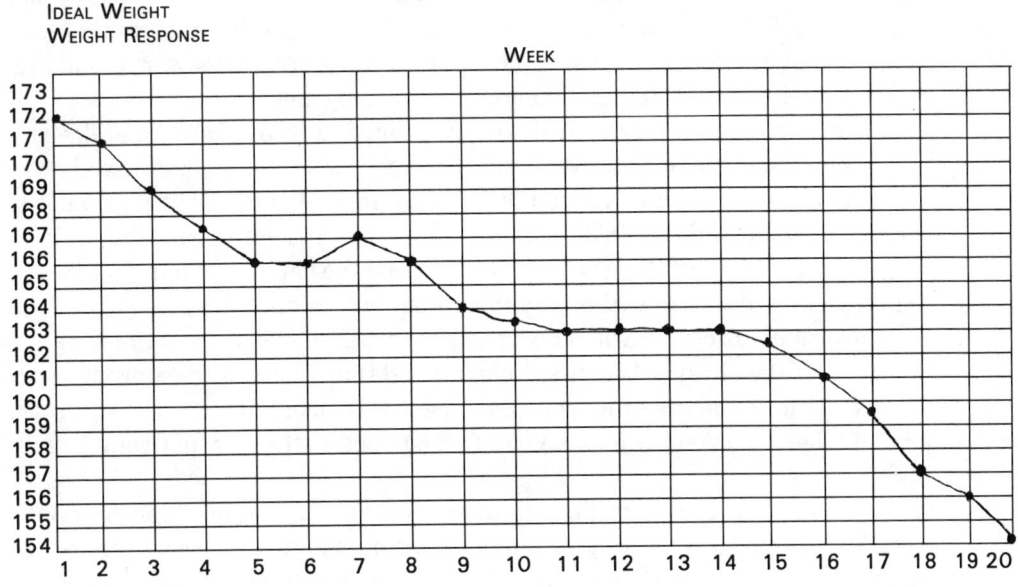

MEASUREMENT RESPONSE

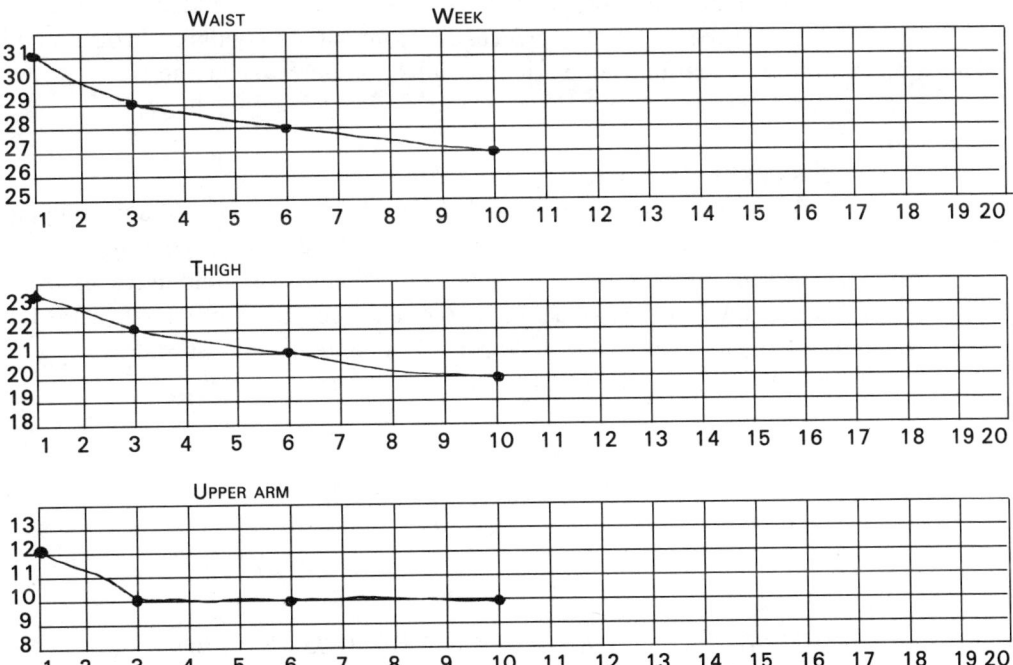

Walking Program

It is now time to make a commitment to begin a walking program. Regular walking is probably the most important aspect of a weight-control program. When you follow a walking program consistently, you realize that you *do* have the power to develop a new habit. This realization gives you power to build the other new habits required in a weight-control program.

Walking is something that almost everyone is able to do. Walking does not require special equipment, a special time, or a special place. If possible walk with a friend; but walk regularly, even if you have to walk alone. At first do not be concerned about walking fast; walk at a pace that is comfortable and pleasant for you. The important thing is for you to develop the habit of walking for twenty minutes every day—or at the very minimum, every other day.

A walking program will do wonders for you. In a very short time you will be aware of the physical benefits. You will find that you have greater vigor and energy. At first you may feel you can't spare the time; but soon you will reach a point where the walk will make you feel so good that you won't want to miss it!

The psychological benefits will be as great as the physical benefits. After several weeks on a walking program, you will feel a good sense of accomplishment. You will feel worthwhile because you have been able to keep a commitment. You will feel pleased with yourself because you will know you are improving your body. You will become more optimistic about life. You will also find that the walk will do much to help relieve the tension of a stressful day.

Maybe you are still not convinced of the value of a walking program. All we can say is "give it a try." Perform Assignment #4 (Walking Program) for one month. No cheating. Follow it faithfully for four weeks and then you will be convinced of its value.

ASSIGNMENT #4. *Walking Program*
For five days of each week walk for twenty minutes without stopping. Continue for four weeks. Keep a record of your progress on Worksheet #4. (A sample worksheet is given on p. 77; blank worksheets are found in Appendix C.) At the end of the first two weeks give yourself a reward for success; after two weeks the benefits of walking will probably be sufficient reward.

WORKSHEET #4. WALKING RECORD SAMPLE

WEEK 1. DATES 5/10-16

DAY	TIME STARTED	TIME ENDED	WITH WHOM	WHERE
Monday	6:30	7:00	Jean & Lois	around the park
Tuesday	6:30	7:05	Jean & Lois	to boat basin
Wednesday	6:35	7:00	Lois	around the park
Thursday	—	—	—	—
Friday	6:30	7:00	Jean & Lois	around the park
Saturday	9:30	10:00	Mindy	to stadium
Sunday	—	—	.	—

WEEK 2. DATES 5/17-23

Monday	7:00	7:30	Jean	around the park
Tuesday	6:30	7:00	Jean & Lois	to Mindy's house
Wednesday	6:30	7:00	Jean & Lois	around the park
Thursday	6:30	7:00	Jean	" "
Friday	—	—	—	—
Saturday	9:00	9:30	Mindy	around the park
Sunday	—	—	—	—

WEEK 3. DATES 5/23-29

Monday	6:30	7:00	Jean & Lois	to boat basin
Tuesday	6:45	7:15	" "	around the park
Wednesday	6:30	7:00	Lois	"
Thursday	6:30	7:00	Jean & Lois	"
Friday	6:30	7:00	Jean & Lois	"
Saturday	9:30	10:00	Mindy	to stadium
Sunday	—	—	—	—

GETTING OFF TO A GOOD START

WEEK 4. DATES 30 – June 5

Monday	6:30	7:00	Jean & Lois	around the park
Tuesday	6:30	7:00	" "	" " "
Wednesday	6:30	7:00	" "	" " "
Thursday	6:30	7:00	" "	" " "
Friday	6:30	7:00	Mindy	" " "
Saturday	9:30	10:00	"	" " "
Sunday	–	–	–	–

REWARD SELECTED Go to a movie ; buy new jogging shoes

REWARDS EARNED AND OBTAINED WHEN May 16, May 23, May 29, June 5
May 22 - movie ; June 4 - new jogging shoes

CHAPTER 9

Getting There

A diet in which the nutrients are balanced is important at any time, but it is especially important when you are restricting the amount of food you eat. For weight-loss diets we recommend a basic 1000-calorie diet for women and a 1500-calorie diet for men. The basic diets are balanced in the nutrients and contain at least the RDA of all the nutrients (except iron for women of childbearing age). We will give you the basic principles of the diets and then you decide what food you wish to eat at each meal.

Food Exchanges

The diets are based upon our food-exchange list, which has been adapted from that developed jointly by the American Diabetes Association and the American Dietetic Association with additional material from the "Nutritive Value of American Foods," Agricultural Handbook no. 456, Washington, D.C.: U.S. GPO, 1975. In the exchange lists foods are grouped according to roughly similar nutrient and caloric values. One exchange of food in a group has about the same number of grams of protein, carbohydrate, and fat as one exchange of another food in the same group. In planning meals one exchange of any food in a group can be traded for one exchange of any other food in that same group. However, an exchange of food in one group cannot be traded for an exchange in another group.

One exchange is a small amount—a portion of a specific food. For example, one small apple or half a small banana or one half of a cup of orange juice constitutes one fruit exchange. Or one large egg or one-quarter cup creamed cottage cheese or 1 oz. ground round constitutes one medium fat exchange. When we speak of an exchange of a certain food, we are referring to the amount that can be exchanged or traded for a certain amount of another food in the same group. Let us consider each exchange group:

Group 1.   Milk Exchanges:

Milk is a good source of protein and the most important source of calcium. (Without milk, or other dairy products, your diet will probably be deficient in calcium, unless you eat a lot of "greens" or soybean products.) Milk is also a good source of riboflavin and vitamin A. For many people fortified milk is their only dietary source of vitamin D. Skim milk contains essentially no fat; low-fat and whole milk contain butterfat, a saturated fat.

You can use milk in many ways in addition to drinking it. An easy way to include extra milk in your diet is to add powdered skim milk to baked goods, casseroles, gravies, and sauces.

Group 2.   Meat Exchanges:

The meat exchange group contains beef, pork, lamb, wild game, cheese, eggs, poultry, fish, and the legumes—dried beans, peas, lentils, peanuts, and soybeans. All of these foods are good sources of protein and many are good sources of zinc, iron, and several of the B-complex vitamins. The foods of animal origin contain vitamin B_{12}, saturated fats, and cholesterol; fish and poultry contain less saturated fat than beef, pork, or lamb. The legumes are good sources of magnesium and potassium, and contain carbohydrate, in addition to protein and unsaturated fat.

The meat group is divided into three subgroups, depending upon the amount of fat present. The animal meat exchanges given in our food-exchange list are based upon a portion of meat that has had all visible fat removed. If the visible fat or meat, and skin of poultry, are not removed, most beef, pork, lamb, game, and poultry would be classed as high-fat meat. If the visible fat is removed, several meat cuts can be classed as low-fat or medium-fat meat exchanges. Poultry with the skin removed is classed as a low-fat exchange.

One animal meat exchange is defined as 1 oz. of cooked meat without bone; 8 oz. of raw meat is approximately equivalent to 6 oz. of cooked meat.

Group 3. Fat Exchanges:

Fats are the most concentrated sources of calories and therefore should be used sparingly. Margarine and butterfats contain vitamin A. Nuts are a good source of protein, as well as of fat. Most fats from vegetable sources contain some essential fatty acids, as well as other mono- and polyunsaturated fats. Hard margarines, although usually prepared from vegetable sources, have been chemically changed to contain mostly saturated fats. Liquids and soft margarines, if prepared from corn, soybean, cottonseed, or safflower oils, are polyunsaturated. Many commercial salad oils are partially hydrogenated. (See Chapter 2 for a discussion of the relationship of fats to heart disease and cancer.)

Group 4. Bread–Cereal–Starchy Vegetable Exchanges:

This group contains all foods made from the various cereal grains such as wheat, oats, rye, and corn, as well as vegetables with a high starch or sugar content. The foods in this group are the most economical source of energy. The vegetables and the whole-grain breads and cereals are good sources of fiber. Whole-grain and enriched flours are good sources of iron and thiamin. The whole grains and vegetables are also good sources of folacin and potassium.

The question is often asked, "Are whole-grain products better than refined-grain products?" To answer this let us consider wheat for an example. A kernel

TABLE 9 NUTRIENT CONTENT OF FLOURS PER 100 GRAMS

	WHOLE WHEAT	WHITE, UNENRICHED	WHITE, ENRICHED
ENERGY, CALORIES	330.0	355.0	355.0
FIBER, CRUDE, GRAMS	2.3	0.3	0.3
LINOLEIC ACID, GRAMS	1.5	0.75	0.75
PROTEIN, GRAMS	13.0	11.0	11.0
VITAMIN B$_6$, MG	0.30	0.05	0.05
CALCIUM, MG	35.0	17.0	17.0
CHROMIUM, MG	0.06	0.02	0.02
VITAMIN E, IU	1.5	0.03	0.03
FLUORIDE, MG	0.1	0.06	0.06
FOLACIN, MG	0.04	0.01	0.01
IRON, MG	3.0	0.6	3.0*
MAGNESIUM, MG	140.0	25.0	25.0
NIACIN, MG	5.0	1.0	5.3*
PANTOTHENIC ACID, MG	1.0	0.5	1.0
PHOSPHORUS, MG	350.0	90.0	90.0
POTASSIUM, MG	400.0	90.0	90.0
RIBOFLAVIN, MG	0.12	0.04	0.4*
THIAMIN, MG	0.5	0.09	0.64*
ZINC, MG	3.0	0.6	—

*Nutrients added to enrich white flour

of wheat consists of a large portion called an *endosperm,* a very small portion called the *germ,* a covering called *bran,* and an outer covering called the *husk.* When flour is refined, everything is removed except the endosperm. Most of the vitamins and minerals and fiber are removed during the refining. Enrichment returns thiamin, niacin, riboflavin, and iron to the flour. However, folacin, vitamin B_6, and other minerals and fiber have not been returned. Table 9 shows the nutrient differences in whole-wheat, enriched white, and unenriched white flour.

Group 5.   Fruit Exchanges:

Fruits are valuable for vitamins, minerals, and fiber. In addition, they are among the most enjoyable of foods. Vitamin C is abundant in citrus fruits and is found in berries and melons. Oranges and cantaloupe are good sources of folacin. The better sources of vitamin A include the yellow fruits, such as apricots and cantaloupes. Most fruits—especially apricots, bananas, berries, grapefruit, cantaloupe, nectarines, oranges, and peaches—are valuable sources of potassium.

Fresh, dried, canned or frozen, and cooked or raw fruits all count as a fruit exchange as long as no sugar is added. (If sugar is added, the amount must be counted as a sugar exchange.) However, see the section on food preparation for a discussion of nutrients retained by various methods.

Group 6.   Vegetable Exchanges:

The foods in this group are the leading sources of many of the vitamins and minerals and fiber, as well as contributing the smallest number of calories of any of the food groups. Dark green and yellow vegetables are among the best sources of vitamin A. Good sources of vitamin C include tomatoes, the cabbage family, green peppers, and greens. High amounts of folacin are found in asparagus, beets, broccoli, brussels sprouts, cauliflower, collards, kale, and lettuce.

Fresh, dried, canned or frozen, and raw or cooked vegetables all count as a vegetable exchange as long as no sugar is added. However, see the section on food preparation for a discussion of the nutrients retained by various methods.

Group 7.   Sugar Exchanges:

We are defining a seventh exchange group, the sugar group. This group includes all natural sugars, such as table sugar, dextrose, fructose, syrups, honey, and molasses. It also includes foods in which sugar is a major ingredient, such as candy and soft drinks. In addition we can include sweet desserts that have a high content of sugar. These foods provide mainly food energy, with a negligible amount of other nutrients.

Group 8. Alcohol Exchanges:

We are also defining an eighth exchange group, the alcohol group. This group includes all of the alcoholic beverages, such as gin, whiskey, rum, vodka, beer, and wines, and any mixtures of alcohol with other foods. Alcoholic beverages provide food energy, but a negligible amount of other nutrients, except for thiamin in beer.

Alcoholic beverages are not recommended, except in small amounts, because alcohol can damage all cells of the body, expecially brain and liver cells.

A modified form of the food-exchange list is given on pp. 84–85. This list is arranged in a condensed form for your convenience. We suggest that you photocopy the list and place it on your refrigerator or a cabinet door so that you can refer to it when you plan your meals. A more comprehensive list is found in Appendix B.

Nonnutrients:

Foods such as black coffee, tea, spices, condiments, and diet drinks contain a negligible amount of food energy or nutrients. However, just because they contain no food energy does not mean they should be used in excess. Coffee, tea, and cola drinks contain caffeine, which is the most widely used drug in the United States. In addition to stimulation of the nervous system, caffeine also causes the kidneys to produce more urine, it stimulates the heart, it dilates the heart's arteries, increases respiration, and relaxes the smooth muscle in the walls of the intestine. Whether or not these effects are detrimental is at present a matter of conjecture. However, wisdom dictates moderation in the use of drinks containing caffeine. Probably the most serious side effect of heavy drinking of coffee or tea or diet drinks is the malnutrition resulting from substituting these beverages for food containing nutrients. This is especially serious for growing children. Pregnant women should not use these drinks because of possible damage to the bone structure of the unborn baby.

Diet drinks frequently contain saccharin, which is considered a mild carcinogen. It is recommended that use should be restricted to not more than 320 mg per day (a diet drink contains 80 mg, and sweetener packages usually contain 30 mg) for an adult and none for nondiabetic children or pregnant women.

A new nonnutritive sweetener, Aspartame, has been approved by the FDA (July 1981). In the future diet drinks may contain Aspartame, which is believed to be safe.

Food Preparation and Preservation

For an exchange diet to be most nutritious, preparation methods that result in the smallest loss of vitamins and minerals should be used. In general, food

FOOD EXCHANGES

MILK EXCHANGE — 8 GRAMS PROTEIN, 12 GRAMS CARBOHYDRATE, 80 CALORIES

SKIM MILK (1 MILK EXCHANGE)
- 1 C SKIM OR NONFAT MILK
- ¼ C POWDERED, REGULAR
- ⅓ C POWDERED, INSTANT
- ½ C EVAPORATED SKIM MILK

LOW-FAT, 2% MILK (1 MILK + 1 FAT)
- 1 C LOW-FAT OR 2% MILK
- 1 C LOW-FAT YOGURT
- 1 C SOYBEAN MILK
- (17% CALCIUM OF COW'S MILK)

WHOLE MILK (1 MILK + 2 FAT)
- 1 C WHOLE MILK
- ½ C EVAPORATED WHOLE MILK
- 1 C MALTED MILK
- 1 C BUTTERMILK

MEAT EXCHANGE — 7 GRAMS PROTEIN, 3 GRAMS FAT, 55 CALORIES
(ALL MEAT HAS HAD ALL SEPARABLE FAT REMOVED AND NONE ADDED IN COOKING.)

LEAN MEAT (1 MEAT EXCHANGE)
1 OZ. MEAT
- FLANK, ROUND, SIRLOIN STEAKS
- BEEF POT ROASTS
- VEAL CUTS EXCEPT BREAST
- CENTER CUT PORK LOIN CHOPS
- LAMB LOIN CHOPS, LEG ROAST
- POULTRY, WITHOUT SKIN
- ALL LIVER, HEART
- ANY FRESH, FROZEN FISH
- ¼ C CANNED TUNA, SALMON
- ¼ C LOW-FAT COTTAGE CHEESE
- 1 OZ. "SLIM" PROCESSED CHEESE
- ½ C COOKED, DRIED LEGUMES
  (1 MEAT + 1 BREAD)

MED.-FAT MEAT (1 MEAT + ½ FAT)
1 OZ. MEAT
- GROUND ROUND, CORNED BEEF
- RIB, CLUB, T-BONE BEEF STEAKS
- BEEF OVEN ROASTS, FRIED LIVER
- BLADE, SHOULDER PORK ROASTS
- BOILED HAM, CANADIAN BACON
- ARM-BLADE LAMB CHOPS
- ¼ C CREAMED COTTAGE CHEESE
- 1 OZ. MOZZARELLA, RICOTTA CHEESE
- 1 WHOLE LARGE EGG
- ½ C COOKED SOYBEANS
- 3½ OZ. TOFU (1 MEAT + 1 BREAD)

HIGH-FAT MEAT (1 MEAT + 1 FAT)
1 OZ. MEAT
- GROUND BEEF, CHUCK, HAMBURGER
- BEEF BRISKET, CORNED BEEF
- VEAL BREAST, STEW MEAT
- PORK SPARERIBS, PICNIC HAM
- GROUND PORK, SALAMI
- COLD CUTS—1 SL., 4½" × ⅛"
- 1 OZ. CHEDDAR, ROQUEFORT, BLUE,
  SWISS, AM. PROCESS CHEESE
- 2 OZ. FRANKFURTERS (1 MEAT + 2½ FAT)
- 2 OZ. SAUSAGE (1 MEAT + 2½ FAT)
- 2 TB. PEANUT BUTTER (1 MEAT + 2 FAT)

BREAD-CEREAL-STARCHY VEGETABLE EXCHANGE — 2 GRAMS PROTEIN, 15 GRAMS CARBOHYDRATE, 70 CALORIES

- 1 SL. BREAD
- 1 PLAIN ROLL
- ½ SM. BAGEL OR MUFFIN
- ½ FRANKFURTER ROLL
- ½ HAMBURGER BUN
- 1 TORTILLA, 6"
- 3 CRACKERS

- ¾ C READY-TO-EAT CEREAL
- ½ C COOKED CEREAL
- ½ C RICE, PASTA, COOKED
- 3 C POPCORN (NO OIL)
- 2½ TB. WHEAT FLOUR
- ¼ C WHEAT GERM
- 2 TB. CORNMEAL

- ½ C COOKED DRIED LEGUMES (+ 1 MEAT)
- ⅓ C CORN, 1 SM. COB
- 1 SM. POTATO, ½ C MASHED POTATOES
- ¾ C PUMPKIN
- ½ C WINTER, ACORN, BUTTERNUT SQUASH
- ¼ C YAM OR SWEET POTATO
- ½ C GREEN PEAS

FRUIT EXCHANGE — 10 GRAMS CARBOHYDRATE, 40 CALORIES

- 1 SM. APPLE, ⅓ C JUICE
- 2 MED. APRICOTS, FRESH, DRIED
- ½ SM. BANANA
- ½ C BERRIES, ¾ C STRAWBERRIES
- 10 LG. CHERRIES

- 2 DATES
- ½ GRAPEFRUIT, ½ C JUICE
- 12 GRAPES, ¼ C JUICE
- ¼ SM. MELON
- 1 SM. ORANGE, ½ C JUICE

- 1 MED. PEACH, PEAR
- ½ C PINEAPPLE, ⅓ C JUICE
- 2 MED. PRUNES, ¼ C JUICE
- 2 TB. RAISINS
- 1 MED. TANGERINE

VEGETABLE EXCHANGE 2 GRAMS PROTEIN, 5 GRAMS CARBOHYDRATE, 25 CALORIES
1 C ANY RAW VEGETABLE, EXCEPT THOSE ON BREAD-CEREAL-STARCHY VEGETABLE LIST
½ C ANY COOKED VEGETABLE, EXCEPT THOSE ON BREAD-CEREAL-STARCHY VEGETABLE LIST
ANY QUANTITY OF RAW: CHINESE CABBAGE, ENDIVE, ESCAROLE, LETTUCE, RADISH, PARSLEY, WATERCRESS

FAT EXCHANGE 5 GRAMS FAT, 45 CALORIES
1 TSP. MARGARINE,** BUTTER, OILS,* MAYONNAISE*
1 TB. SALAD DRESSING,* CREAM CHEESE, 2 TB. CREAM
6 NUTS,* 5 SM. OLIVES,* ⅛ AVOCADO,* 1 STRIP BACON

SUGAR EXCHANGE 12 GRAMS CARBOHYDRATE, 48 CALORIES
1 TB. GRANULATED, BROWN, SUGAR; SYRUPS, JAM
2 TSP. HONEY, 4 TSP. POWDERED SUGAR
¼ OZ. HARD CANDY, 4 OZ. SOFT DRINKS

ALCOHOL EXCHANGE 0–4 GRAMS CARBOHYDRATE, 4–5 GRAMS ALCOHOL, APPROX. 50 CALORIES
4 FL. OZ. BEER   1 FL. OZ. DESSERT WINES   1½ FL. OZ. TABLE WINES   ½ FL. OZ. WHISKEY, RUM, GIN

NONNUTRIENTS: BLACK COFFEE, TEA, SPICES, CONDIMENTS, DIET DRINKS

*Unsaturated fats
**Unsaturated if made from partially hydrogenated seed oils

preparation methods that utilize the lowest heat for the shortest time and the smallest amount of water will preserve the most vitamins. Vitamin C is most easily destroyed by heat, but prolonged cooking will destroy a large percentage of all vitamins. The water-soluble vitamins are also lost in the cooking water, if that water is discarded. The mineral content of a food is not affected by the method, but many minerals are soluble in water and hence are lost if the water is discarded.

High-temperature cooking makes the protein in eggs less easily digested; but eventually all the amino acids are available to the body. But eggs are best when cooked at lower temperatures—boiling water or lower. High temperatures can be destructive to unsaturated fatty acids, causing them to form breakdown products, some of which are destructive to body cells, and may also be carcinogenic. Prolonged heating also changes the structure of unsaturated fatty acids from the natural form to the unnatural form. Oils, such as those used in deep-fat frying, should not be heated over and over.

One of the greatest problems with preparation methods, both commercial and home, is the amount of salt added to the food. As we mentioned in Chapter 2, for people who have a genetic predisposition to hypertension, excess sodium in the diet is implicated as a cause of hypertension. Large amounts of salt are routinely added to prepared foods. For example, fresh peas when boiled and drained contain about 1 mg of sodium per 100 grams of peas. Home-canned peas that are boiled and drained contain about 236 mg sodium per 100 grams; commercially canned peas that are boiled and drained contain about 236 mg sodium per 100 grams of peas. Commercially frozen peas, which are then boiled and drained, contain about 115 mg sodium. The advantage of home cooking over commercial preparation methods is that when you cook fresh peas you can decide how much salt to add.

A problem with commercially and home-canned fruit and frozen fruit is the excessive amount of sugar that is added. When buying canned fruit, it is best to purchase fruit canned in its own juice, without added sugar. If such fruit is not available, buy fruit canned in light syrup and then pour off the syrup before serving the fruit. However, some of the vitamins and minerals will be lost in the syrup.

When possible, fruit should be eaten fresh and raw. When this is not possible because of prohibitive cost of fruit out of season, frozen fruits are the next best choice. However, canned fruits are better than no fruit at all (or better than a rich dessert).

In preparing meat remove all visible fat from the meat before eating it. When buying meat avoid the highly marbled cuts. Avoid cooking methods, such as frying in fat, that add fat to the cooked meat. Poultry should be cooked with the skin on to preserve the moisture; however the skin (which contains most of the fat) should be removed prior to eating the meat.

Meal Planning with Exchange Diets

The basic exchange diets and the exchange lists will enable you to plan your meals using a wide variety of foods without having to calculate calories or nutrients. Table 10 on p. 88 gives our basic exchange diets for weight reduction. These diets were designed with the Senate dietary goals in mind. The nutrient composition given is based upon the average composition of foods within each group in order to obtain the average amount of nutrients.

For the 1000-calorie exchange diet we give you two plans of similar nutrient composition: A, for those who prefer more fruits and vegetables, and B, for those who prefer more breads and starchy vegetables. The diets supply the RDA of all nutrients except iron for women under fifty. Additional iron can be obtained by selecting liver, meat, eggs, legumes, green leafy vegetables, and dried fruits. We recommend an iron supplement for women since it is difficult to obtain 18-mg iron from the usual foods selected on a calorie-restricted diet.

For men we recommend a 1500-calorie exchange diet. This diet supplies the RDA for all nutrients for men. (Niacin appears low; this is due to the fact that the RDA includes the niacin that can be made from the protein in the diet.)

We recommend, for both men and women, that two thirds of your fat exchanges be obtained from foods that contain unsaturated fatty acids. These foods are marked with an (*) on the exchange list. We also recommend a daily multivitamin and multimineral supplement plus 500 mg of vitamin C.

Although our basic exchange diets are balanced to give you the needed nutrients, you might not choose a sufficient variety of foods to give you the RDA of all nutrients. Also the RDA is designed for all healthy persons, but it does not take into account additional stress on your body which may be caused by a reduced-calorie diet.

You will also note that there are no sugar or alcohol exchanges allowed on the basic restricted-calorie diets. On such diets you must be very careful to obtain a balance of the essential nutrients; you cannot afford to eat food that contains food energy and nothing else. These foods we call "empty-calorie" or "extra-fuel" foods. If you must eat some empty-calorie foods, it is better to eat them in addition to your basic diet and to treat them as extra-fuel foods. (Later in this chapter we will explain how to handle extra-fuel foods.)

Nonnutritive sweeteners, such as those found in diet drinks, do not contribute any food energy to your diet. However, for two reasons we do not recommend an unlimited use of these sweeteners. First there is evidence that the saccharin in these sweeteners may be dangerous to your health. (See discussion under "Nonnutrients.") The second reason is that as you progress in our weight-control program, you will lose your craving for sweets. The nonnutritive sweeteners just prolong this craving. We believe it is better for you to gradually cut

TABLE 10   BASIC EXCHANGE DIETS FOR WEIGHT REDUCTION

FOR WOMEN: 1000 CALORIE

EXCHANGES	CAL	PRO GRAMS	CHO GRAMS	FAT GRAMS	CA MG	IRON MG	VIT. A IU	THIA MG	RIB MG	NIA MG	VIT. C MG
PLAN A											
2 MILK	160	16	24	—	684	0.2	208	0.18	0.88	0.48	4
5 MEAT	275	35	—	15	150	4.5	200	0.45	0.50	6.50	2
4 FRUIT	160	—	40	—	52	2.0	2452	0.16	0.12	1.44	72
3 VEG.	75	6	15	—	114	1.8	4446	0.15	0.24	1.47	69
3 BREAD	210	6	45	—	57	2.7	1320	0.24	0.18	2.37	9
3 FAT	135	—	—	15	*	*	*	*	*	*	*
TOTALS	1015	63	124	30	1057	11.2	8626	1.16	1.92	12.26	156
RDA	N	44	N	N	800	18.0	4000	1.0	1.2	13.0	60

25% PRO   49% CHO   27% FAT

EXCHANGES	CAL	PRO GRAMS	CHO GRAMS	FAT GRAMS	CA MG	IRON MG	VIT. A IU	THIA MG	RIB MG	NIA MG	VIT. C MG
PLAN B											
2 MILK	160	16	24	—	684	0.2	208	0.18	0.88	0.48	4
5 MEAT	275	35	—	15	150	4.5	200	0.45	0.50	6.50	2
3 FRUIT	120	—	30	—	39	1.5	1839	0.12	0.09	1.08	54
2 VEG.	50	4	10	—	76	1.2	2964	0.10	0.16	0.98	46
4 BREAD	280	8	60	—	76	3.6	1760	0.32	0.24	3.16	12
3 FAT	135	—	—	15	*	*	*	*	*	*	*
TOTALS	1020	63	124	30	1025	11.0	6971	1.17	1.87	12.22	118
RDA		44			800	18.0	4000	1.0	1.2	13.0	60

25% PRO   49% CHO   27% FAT

FOR MEN: 1500 CALORIE

EXCHANGES	CAL	PRO	CHO	FAT	CA	IRON	VIT. A	THIA	RIB	NIA	VIT. C
2 MILK	160	16	24	—	684	0.2	208	0.18	0.88	0.48	4
5 MEAT	275	35	—	15	150	4.5	200	0.45	0.50	6.50	2
4 FRUIT	160	—	40	—	52	2.0	2452	0.16	0.12	1.44	72
3 VEG.	75	6	15	—	114	1.8	4446	0.15	0.24	1.47	69
8 BREAD	560	16	120	—	152	7.2	3520	0.64	0.48	6.32	24
6 FAT	270	—	—	30	*	*	*	*	*	*	*
TOTALS	1500	73	199	45	1152	15.7	10826	1.58	2.22	16.21	171
RDA		56			800	10.0	5000	1.4	1.6	18.0	60

20% PRO   53% CHO   27% FAT

ABBREVIATIONS:
CAL   CALORIES   CA   CALCIUM   RIB   RIBOFLAVIN
PRO   PROTEIN   VIT. A VITAMIN A   NIA   NIACIN
CHO   CARBOHYDRATE   THIA   THIAMIN   VIT. C VITAMIN C

*Fat exchanges, except for nuts and avocado, have essentially zero quantities of these nutrients.

down on the amount of sugar that you use rather than substitute nonnutritive sweeteners. For example, use fruit juices with less and less (or no) added sugar instead of soft drinks. You can also use club soda or plain water when you want something to drink.

We also recommend that you decrease the amount of salt that you use, even though salt does not contribute any food energy to your diet. As we explained in Chapter 2, a high salt intake is implicated as a possible cause of high blood pressure for those who are genetically predisposed. The Senate Select Committee on Nutrition and Human Needs has recommended reducing your salt intake to about 5 grams per day. You can achieve this reduction by removing the salt shaker from the table and by not eating salty processed foods and condiments.

To plan your meals for the day select one of the basic exchange diets given on p. 88, and divide the number of exchanges into three meals. Research results are mixed concerning the value of more than three meals a day. Some research indicates that six meals are more conducive to weight loss than three meals. However, other research has indicated that building a habit of eating only three times a day helps break the snacking habit, and hence leads to a life-style more conducive to maintaining weight loss. You must decide whether a three- or six-meal plan is best for you.

With the basic exchange diets and the exchange list how do you plan meals for yourself and your family? Let us follow through the procedure in some detail:

Jean has selected the 1000-calorie, Plan A, exchange diet. For the first day she decides on the following meal distribution:

Total: 2 milk, 5 meat, 3 fat, 3 bread, 4 fruit, 3 veg.
Breakfast: 1 milk, 1 meat, 1 fat, 1 bread, 2 fruit
Lunch: 1 milk, 1 meat, 1 fat, 1 bread, 1 fruit, 1 veg.
Dinner: 3 meat, 1 fat, 1 bread, 1 fruit, 2 veg.

For breakfast Jean decides on milk, eggs, toast, and orange juice. She decides to drink skim milk so she can use her fat exchange for butter on her toast. She also decides to save her second fruit exchange for her morning break. For lunch Jean mixes 1 tsp mayonnaise with ¼ cup tuna and ½ cup chopped celery, and puts it on a lettuce leaf on 1 slice whole-wheat bread. This takes care of her meat, fat, bread, and vegetable exchanges. For her afternoon break she has 8 oz. plain yogurt in which she mixes 1 small pear. This accounts for her milk and fruit exchanges. For dinner Jean decides to have veal cutlets with potatoes, summer squash, and a tossed green salad with dressing. She saves her fruit to eat just before bedtime. Her meal plan looks like this:

Breakfast	Lunch	Dinner
8 OZ. SKIM MILK—1 MILK	¼ C TUNA—1 MEAT	3 OZ. VEAL CUTLETS—3 MEAT
1 EGG—1 MEAT, ½ FAT	1 TSP. MAYONNAISE—1 FAT	1 SM. POTATO—1 BREAD
1 SL. WW TOAST—1 BREAD	½ C CELERY, LETTUCE—1 VEG.	½ C SUMMER SQUASH—1 VEG.
½ TSP. BUTTER—½ FAT	1 SL. WW. BREAD—1 BREAD	1 C TOSSED GREEN SALAD—1
½ C ORANGE JUICE—1 FRUIT		VEG.
		1 TB. SALAD DRESSING—1 FAT

Snack	Snack	Snack
2 APRICOTS—1 FRUIT	8 OZ. PLAIN SKIM MILK YOGURT—	¼ SM. HONEYDEW MELON—1 FRUIT
	1 MILK	
	1 SM. PEAR—1 FRUIT	

FOR HER SECOND DAY, JEAN DECIDES ON THE FOLLOWING DISTRIBUTION AND MEAL PLAN:

> BREAKFAST: 1 MILK, 1 BREAD, 2 FRUIT
> LUNCH: ½ MILK, 2 MEAT, 1 FRUIT, 1 VEG.
> DINNER: ½ MILK, 3 MEAT, 3 FAT, 2 BREAD, 1 FRUIT, 2 VEG.

Breakfast	Lunch	Dinner
½ C OATMEAL—1 BREAD	2 OZ. CHICKEN DRUMSTICKS,	3 OZ. HAMBURGER—3 MEAT, 3 FAT
2 TB. RAISINS—1 FRUIT	NO SKIN—2 MEAT	½ C RICE—1 BREAD
½ C SKIM MILK—½ MILK	2 SM. TOMATOES—1 VEG.	⅓ C CORN—1 BREAD
½ GRAPEFRUIT—1 FRUIT	½ C SKIM MILK—½ MILK	½ C GREEN BEANS—1 VEG.
		CARROT STICKS—1 VEG.

Snack	Snack	Snack
½ C SKIM MILK—½ MILK	1 SM. APPLE—1 FRUIT	½ C SKIM MILK—½ MILK
		½ SM. BANANA—1 FRUIT

You will note that you do not have to count calories, or grams of carbohydrate; this has all been done for you. All you need to do is decide how you will distribute your total exchanges throughout the day; then decide what foods in each exchange list you will eat that day. As you plan for the right number of exchanges, your calories and nutrients will be planned for simultaneously.

It is very easy to adapt your meal plans to nondieting members of your family. You need only give them a larger quantity of each of the foods in your meal plan. You can then be assured that your family will also have balanced, nutritious meals.

Pages 89, 98, and 99 give sample meal plans for each of the basic exchange diets. These plans also show you how to account for the number of exchanges of each food group so that you can be sure you have the right number of exchanges.

One important principle in planning your meals is to use all of the allowed exchanges. "Experienced" dieters, who are used to crash diets, think they are eating too much food. They aren't. These basic diets are designed for you to lose one and a half to two pounds per week—and feel good while you are doing it.

ASSIGNMENT 5A: *Meal Planning:*

Using the meal-planning forms in Appendix C, plan your meals for a week. Account for the number of exchanges of each food group each day. Plan your meals with foods that are available and that you like. Do not use any sugar exchanges. Do not substitute foods in one group for foods in another food group.

ASSIGNMENT 5B. *Following Your Meal Plan:*

Follow your meal plan for one week. Check off each food as you eat it. Do not substitute foods unless an emergency arises. Substitute only with another food in the same exchange group. When you follow your meal plan for a week, give yourself a nice reward.

Continue planning your meals using the planning forms in Appendix C for another five weeks. Give yourself a nice reward for each week that you follow your plan. Continue planning your meals using the basic exchange diets until you reach your desired body weight.

What if you "blow" your meal plan for a day? Perhaps you went out for lunch with a friend and "pigged out." Maybe the boss invited you to dinner and there was nothing to eat except fats and sweets. What do you do after you have blown your plan for a day? Nothing. You need not feel guilty or upset. A balanced diet will not be destroyed by one day out of kilter. Just go back to your meal plan the next day. After you have followed your meal plans for several weeks, you will know how to select foods for special occasions.

However, to help you at the moment, here are some suggestions to follow when you eat out at restaurants, snack bars, or friends' homes:

RESTAURANTS

1. Eat lightly during the day so you will have some exchanges left for your eating time out.
2. Select low-calorie appetizers such as relishes, tomato juice, broth, or tossed salad; leave the rolls.
3. Trim off all excess fat from meats; leave the gravies.
4. Remove the skin from poultry and breading from fish.
5. Order plain foods; avoid cream sauces, gravies, breading, and fried foods.
6. Order dressings and salad dressing on the side, so you can control the amount you use.
7. Feel free to order your food exactly as you want it.
8. If the restaurant serves smörgåsbord style, fill your plate with salads before you get to the other foods.

WORKSHEET #5. MEAL-PLANNING RECORD   NAME _____

Sample, 1000 calorie, plan A

DAY	BREAKFAST 1 MILK, 1 MEAT, 1 FAT 1 BREAD, 1 FRUIT	LUNCH 1 MILK, 1 MEAT, 1 FAT 1 BREAD, 2 FRUIT, 1 VEG.	DINNER 0 MILK, 3 MEAT, 1 FAT 1 BREAD, 1 FRUIT, 2 VEG.	TOTAL EXCHANGES 2 MILK, 5 MEAT, 3 FAT 3 BREAD, 4 FRUIT, 3 VEG.
SUNDAY 5/12	1 cup skim milk - 1 milk 1 boiled egg - 1 meat & fat 1 sl. whole wheat toast - 1 bread 1 tsp margarine - 1 fat ½ c. orange juice - 1 fruit	1 c. beef bouillon - ½ meat 3 rye wafers - 1 bread celery sticks - 1 veg 1 c. peach slices - ½ fruit 1 c. skim milk buttermilk - 1 milk	3 oz broiled veal steaks - 3 meat ½ c. gr. beans - 1 veg lettuce-tomato salad - 1 veg 1 tb Italian dressing - 1 fat 1 potato - 1 bread 1 c. fruit compote - 1 fruit	MILK 2 MEAT 4½ FAT 3 BREAD 3 FRUIT 4 VEG. 3
MONDAY 5/13	1½ c. skim milk - 1½ milk ½ c. oatmeal - 1 bread 2 tb. raisins - 1 fruit 1 c. pineapple juice - 1 fruit	2 oz Chicken breast - 2 meat ½ c. rice w. parsley - 1 bread ½ tsp margarine - ½ fat radishes - 1 veg ½ c. skim milk - ½ milk ½ c. banana - 1 fruit	3 oz ground round - 3 meat & fat 1 c. tossed salad - 1 veg ½ c. green beans - 1 veg 2 tb. sour cream - 1 fat 1 potato - 1 bread ½ c. cantaloupe - 1 fruit	MILK 2 MEAT 5 FAT 3 BREAD 3 FRUIT 4 VEG. 3
TUESDAY 5/14	1 c. skim milk - 1 milk 1 sl. French toast - 1 bread, 1 meat, ½ fat orange sections - 1 fruit	¼ c. cottage cheese - 1 meat ½ c. pineapple - 1 fruit lettuce - 1 veg 1 cob corn - 1 bread ½ tsp margarine - ½ fat ¾ cup strawberries - 1 fruit	3 oz pork roast - 3 meat, 1½ fat 1 c. green salad - 1 veg carrot sticks - 1 veg ½ tb French dressing - ½ fat ½ cup squash - 1 bread 1 large pear - 2 fruit	MILK 2 MEAT 5 FAT 3 BREAD 3 FRUIT 4 VEG. 3

WEDNESDAY 5/15

1 cup skim milk - 1 milk
Baked eggs on toast - 1 meat, 1 bread, ½ fat
½ grapefruit - 1 fruit
12 grapes - 1 fruit

½ c tuna - 1 meat
1 sl ww bread - 1 bread
1 tsp mayonnaise - 1 fat
½ c. chopped celery, 1 tomato - 1 veg
3/4 c. strawberries - 1 fruit

3 oz lamb roast - 3 meat
Sauteed green pepper - 1 veg, 1 fat
½ c. curried brown rice - 1 bread
1 c. skim milk - 1 milk
½ c. zucchini - 1 veg
2 med. plums - 1 fruit

MILK 2
MEAT 5
FAT 1½
BREAD 3
FRUIT 4
VEG. 3

THURSDAY 5/16

1 c skim milk - 1 milk
1 fluffy omelette - 1 meat, 1 fat
1 sl ww toast - 1 bread
½ tsp margarine - ½ fat
½ c. orange juice - 1 fruit

1 oz chicken livers - 1 meat, 1 veg
½ c. mushrooms - 1 veg
½ c noodles - 1 bread
lettuce wedge - 1 veg
1 tb. French dressing - ½ fat
½ c fruit cocktail - 1 fruit
1 c skim milk - 1 milk

3 oz roast chicken - 3 meat
1 sm tomato - 1 veg
½ c peas & onions - ½ veg, ½ br.
1 potato w. parsley - 1 bread
1 tsp margarine - 1 fat
½ c. cherries - 1 fruit

MILK 2
MEAT 5
FAT 3
BREAD 3½
FRUIT 3
VEG. 3½

FRIDAY 5/17

1 c. skim milk - 1 milk
1 boiled egg - 1 meat, 1 fat
½ muffin - 1 bread
½ tsp margarine - ½ fat
1 tangerine - 1 fruit

2 oz sole - 1 meat
½ c. rice - 1 bread
1 tsp margarine - 1 fat
celery & carrot sticks - 1 veg
1 c skim milk - 1 milk
3/4 c papaya - 1 fruit

2 oz ground round - 2 meat, 1 fat
½ c. mashed potatoes - 1 bread
½ c. cooked carrots - 1 veg
½ c. cooked beets - 1 veg
½ c. raspberries - 1 fruit

MILK 2
MEAT 5
FAT 3
BREAD 3
FRUIT 4
VEG. 3

SATURDAY 5/18

1 c. skim milk - 1 milk
3/4 c. cereal - 1 bread
½ c. orange juice - 1 fruit
½ c. stewed prunes - 1 fruit

1 c. skim milk - 1 milk
1 sl. ww bread - 1 bread
1 oz cheddar cheese - 1 meat, 1 fat
lettuce - 1 veg
1 tsp mayonnaise - 1 fat
1 large apple - 2 fruit

4 oz salmon steak - 4 meat
lemon wedge
1 tsp margarine - 1 fat
½ c. rice - 1 bread
½ c. mushrooms - 1 veg
1 c. greek salad - 1 veg
1 sl. watermelon - 1 fruit

MILK 2
MEAT 5
FAT 3
BREAD 3
FRUIT 4
VEG. 3

WORKSHEET #5. MEAL-PLANNING RECORD   NAME_____

Sample, 1000 calorie, Plan B   Week of March 10-16

DAY	BREAKFAST 1 MILK, 1 MEAT, 1 FAT 1 BREAD, 1 FRUIT	LUNCH 1 MILK, 1 MEAT, 1 FAT 1 BREAD, 2 FRUIT, 1 VEG.	DINNER 0 MILK, 3 MEAT, 1 FAT 1 BREAD, 1 FRUIT, 2 VEG.	TOTAL EXCHANGES 2 MILK, 5 MEAT, 3 FAT 3 BREAD, 4 FRUIT, 3 VEG.
SUNDAY 3/10	1 c. skim milk - 1 milk 1 boiled egg - 1 meat, ½ fat 1 slice toast - 1 bread 2 plums - 1 fruit	1 c. skim milk - 1 milk Grilled cheese sandwich 2 sl bread - 2 bread 1 oz cheese - 1 meat, 1 fat 1 sm apple - 1 fruit	2 oz ham - 2 meat, 2 fat ½ c. peas - 1 veg ½ c. Hubbard squash - 1 bread ½ c. lettuce-tomato salad - 1 veg 1 orange - 1 fruit	MILK 2 MEAT 4 FAT 3½ BREAD 4 FRUIT 4 VEG. 2
MONDAY 3/11	1 c. skim milk - 1 milk 1 sl. toast - 1 bread ½ tsp margarine - ½ fat 1 boiled egg - 1 meat, ½ fat 2 plums - 1 fruit	½ c. lowfat cottage cheese - 1 meat 1 orange - 1 fruit 2 graham crackers - 1 bread 1 c. skim milk - 1 milk	3 oz mackerel - 3 meat ⅔ c rice - 1 bread 1 tsp margarine - 1 fat ½ c. mixed veg - 1 veg 1 c. lettuce - 1 tb dressing - 1 fat ½ c. raspberries - 1 fruit	MILK 2 MEAT 5 FAT 3 BREAD 3 FRUIT 3 VEG. 2
TUESDAY 3/12	1 c. skim milk - 1 milk 1 poached egg - 1 meat, ½ fat 1 sl. toast - 1 bread ½ c. orange juice - 1 fruit	1 c. skim milk - 1 milk 1 sl. bread - 1 bread 2 oz tuna - 1 meat lettuce wedge - 1 veg 1 tsp mayonnaise - 1 fat 1 apple - 1 fruit	3 oz ground round - 3 meat 1½ fat 1 sm. potato - 2 bread ½ c. green beans - 1 veg 4 slices peaches - 1 fruit	MILK 2 MEAT 5 FAT 4 BREAD 3 FRUIT 3 VEG. 2

WEDNESDAY 3/13

3/4 c. cereal - 1 bread
1 c. skim milk - 1 milk
1 oz. chicken - 1 meat
1 sl. toast - 1 bread
1 tsp margarine - 1 fat

1 sl. bread - 1 bread
1 sl. cheddar cheese - 1 meat &
  1 fat
1 carrot - 1 veg
1 peach - 1 fruit
1/2 c. orange juice - 1 fruit

3 oz. very lean steak - 3 meat
  1 fat
1/2 c. rice - 1 bread
1/2 c. green beans - 1 veg
1 c. skim milk - 1 milk
1 apple - 1 fruit

MILK 2
MEAT 5
FAT 3
BREAD 3
FRUIT 3
VEG. 2

THURSDAY 3/14

1 c. 2% milk - 1 milk & 1 fat
1 scrambled egg - 1 meat w/ 1 fat
1 sl. toast - 1 bread
1/2 grapefruit - 1 fruit

1 c. lowfat cottage cheese -
  2 meat
1/2 c. rice -
1 tomato - 1 veg
1/2 c. pears - 1 fruit
1 c. skim milk - 1 milk

2 drumsticks - 2 meat
1/2 c. cabbage - 1 veg
1 c. lettuce & tomato - 1 veg
1 tb. French dressing - 1 fat
1 large potato - 2 bread
1 pear - 1 fruit

MILK 2
MEAT 5
FAT 3
BREAD 4
FRUIT 3
VEG. 3

FRIDAY 3/15

1 c. skim milk - 1 milk
1 sl. toast - 1 bread
1 tsp. butter - 1 fat
1/2 c. grapefruit juice - 1 fruit
1 boiled egg - 1 meat w/ 1 fat

1/4 c. tuna - 1 meat
5 saltine crackers - 1 bread
1 c. skim milk - 1 milk
1 apple - 1 fruit

1/2 c. spaghetti - 1 bread
3 oz. ground round - 3 meat + 1/2 fat
tomatoes onions - 1 veg
1 cucumber - 1 veg
1 c. strawberries - 1 fruit

MILK 2
MEAT 5
FAT 3
BREAD 3
FRUIT 3
VEG. 2

SATURDAY 3/16

1 poached egg - 1 meat & 1/2 fat
1 sl. toast - 1 bread
1 tsp margarine - 1 fat
1 c. skim milk - 1 milk
1/2 c. orange juice - 1 fruit

1/4 c. tuna - 1 meat
5 saltine crackers - 1 bread
1 c. lettuce - 1 veg
1/2 c. cherries - 1 fruit
1 c. skim milk - 1 milk

3 oz. lean steak - 1 meat w/ 1/2 fat
1/2 c. asparagus - 1 veg
1 small potato - 1 bread
1/2 c. corn - 1 bread
1/2 c. cherries - 1 fruit

MILK 2
MEAT 5
FAT 3
BREAD 4
FRUIT 3
VEG. 2

WORKSHEET #5. MEAL-PLANNING RECORD   NAME _____

Sample, 1500 calorie   Week of April 17-23.

DAY	BREAKFAST 1 MILK, 1 MEAT, 1 FAT 1 BREAD, 1 FRUIT	LUNCH 1 MILK, 1 MEAT, 1 FAT 1 BREAD, 2 FRUIT, 1 VEG.	DINNER 0 MILK, 3 MEAT, 1 FAT 1 BREAD, 1 FRUIT, 2 VEG.	TOTAL EXCHANGES 2 MILK, 5 MEAT, 3 FAT 3 BREAD, 4 FRUIT, 3 VEG.
SUNDAY 4/17	1 c. skim milk - 1 milk 1 c. cooked cereal - 2 bread 1 muffin - 2 bread ½ grapefruit - 1 fruit	1 c. skim milk - 1 milk 2 sl. bread - 2 bread 2 oz cold cuts - 2 meat + 2 fat 1 carrot - 1 veg 1 banana - 2 fruit	3 oz roast beef - 3 meat, 3 fat 1½ c. potato - 2 bread ½ c. green beans - 1 veg 1 tomato - 1 veg 1 pc. watermelon - 1 fruit	MILK 2 MEAT 5 FAT 5 BREAD 8 FRUIT 4 VEG 3
MONDAY 4/18	1 c. skim milk - 1 milk 1 boiled egg - 1 meat, ½ fat 2 sl. toast - 2 bread ½ tsp. margarine - ½ fat ½ c. orange juice - 1 fruit	1 c. skim milk - 1 milk 2 sl. bread - 2 bread ½ c. tuna - 2 meat 2 tsp. mayonnaise - 2 fat celery sticks - 1 veg 1 large apple - 2 fruit	2 c. beans + rice, ½ c. mushroom - 4 bread, 2 fat, 2 meat, 1 veg 1 c. tossed green salad - 1 veg ½ Tb Italian dressing - 1 fat ¾ c. strawberries - 1 fruit	MILK 2 MEAT 5 FAT 5 BREAD 8 FRUIT 4 VEG 3
TUESDAY 4/19	1 c. skim milk - 1 milk 1 c. cooked cereal - 2 bread ½ c. pineapple juice - 1 fruit 1 tsp margarine - 1 fat	1 c. skim milk - 1 milk 2 sl. bread - 2 bread 2 tsp. margarine - 2 fat 2 oz chicken w/o skin - 2 meat 1 carrot - 1 veg 1 large orange - 2 fruit	3 oz. veal cutlets - 3 meat 1 c. mashed potatoes - 3 bread 2 tsp margarine - 2 fat ½ c. peas - 1 bread ½ c. carrots - 2 veg 1 pc watermelon - 1 fruit	MILK 2 MEAT 5 FAT 5 BREAD 8 FRUIT 4 VEG 3
WEDNESDAY 4/20	1 c. skim milk - 1 milk 1 boiled egg - 1 meat, ½ fat 2 sl. toast - 2 bread ½ c. orange juice - 1 fruit.	1 c. skim milk - 1 milk 2 sl. bread - 2 bread ½ c. tuna - 2 meat ½ Tb dressing - ½ fat 4 oz veg juice - 1 veg 1 large apple - 2 fruit	1 burrito - 2 meat, 4 bread, 2 fat lettuce wedge - 1 veg ½ Tb salad dressing - ½ fat ½ c. summer squash - 1 veg 1 c. raspberries - 2 fruit	MILK 2 MEAT 5 FAT 3½ BREAD 8 FRUIT 4 VEG 3

THURSDAY 4/21

1 c. skim milk - 1 milk
1 c. cooked cereal - 2 bread
½ grapefruit - 1 fruit

1 c. yogurt - 1 meat
¾ c. strawberries - 1 fruit
2 sl. ww bread - 1 bread
1 tsp margarine - 1 fat
2 sl. cheese - 2 meat, 2 fat
1 carrot - 1 veg
1 apple - 1 fruit

3 oz ground round - 3 meat, 1½ fat
1 c. mashed potatoes - 2 bread
½ tsp margarine - ½ fat
1 c. green beans - 2 veg
½ c. corn - 1 bread
1 c. raspberries - 2 fruit

MILK 2
MEAT 5
FAT 5
BREAD 7
FRUIT 4
VEG. 3

FRIDAY 4/22

1 c. skim milk - 1 milk
1 scrambled egg - 1 meat, 1 fat
2 sl. toast - 2 bread
½ c. orange juice - 1 fruit

1 c. skim milk - 1 milk
2 sl. bread - 2 bread
2 sl. cold cuts - 2 meat, 2 fat
4 oz veg. juice - 1 veg
1 large apple - 2 fruit

3 oz roast chicken, no skin - 3 meat
1 c. mashed potato - 2 bread
1 c. cooked cabbage - 2 veg
1 c. green peas - 2 bread
½ cantaloupe - 2 fruit

MILK 2
MEAT 6
FAT 3
BREAD 8
FRUIT 5
VEG. 3

SATURDAY 4/23

1 c. skim milk - 1 milk
1 c. cooked cereal - 2 bread
1 grapefruit - 2 fruit

1 c. yogurt - 1 milk
¾ c. strawberries - 1 fruit
2 frankfurters - 2 med, 2 fat
2 buns - 4 bread
1 c. cooked greens - 2 veg
½ Tb Italian dressing - ½ fat

3 oz. ground round - 3 meat, 1½ fat
1 c. spaghetti - 2 bread
1 c. tomatoes, onions - 2 veg
½ c. cantaloupe - 2 fruit

MILK 2
MEAT 5
FAT 4
BREAD 8
FRUIT 5
VEG. 4

SNACK BAR, FAST-FOOD PLACES, CAFETERIAS, ETC.

1. Select plain soda or water or milk instead of colas or milkshakes.
2. Ask for the smallest serving possible because most places do not serve low-calorie foods.
3. Ask for open-face sandwiches without dressings.
4. If breaded fish or fried chicken is available, order and then remove the breading or skin and you will have a reasonably low-calorie meat. (Granted, there won't be much left.)
5. Plain hamburgers, tacos, and tostadas are lowest in calories and fat of the fast-food items.
6. Make your own salad from a salad bar if available.
7. At a cafeteria decide *before* you get into line what you will order.

AT A FRIEND'S OR A BANQUET

1. If possible mostly fill your plate with raw vegetables.
2. Eat very slowly; spend as much time as possible talking and listening.
3. Graciously refuse seconds by saying, "I already have some, thank you."

You may have noticed that the foods on the exchange lists are mainly simple, plain foods rather than dishes like casseroles and soups or other mixtures. It is much easier for a beginner on the program to stick with the simple foods. However, a very important part of this program is that it permits you to eat with your family and to eat your favorite foods. Suppose your family likes soups, casseroles, and other one-dish meals. What then? No problem. It is only necessary for you to determine the number of exchanges of each food group for one serving of the food. How is this done? Let us take a few examples to show you how to determine the exchanges in any recipe. To determine the exchanges per serving, you need only total the exchanges for the whole recipe and divide that number by the number of servings in the recipe. It is important, however, for you to measure the serving size carefully. Let us take some recipes and determine the exchanges per serving:

CHOW MEIN (SERVES 8)

8 OZ. DICED PORK—*6 meat, 6 fat
8 OZ. DICED VEAL—6 meat, 3 fat
8 OZ. DICED BEEF—6 meat, 6 fat
3 TB. SOY SAUCE—0
1 CUP WATER—0
1 C DICED CELERY—1 veg.
2 TB. CORNSTARCH—1 bread
10 OZ. WATER CHESTNUTS—2 veg.
2½ C BEAN SPROUTS—2½ veg.
2 OZ. MUSHROOMS—1 veg.
8 C COOKED RICE—16 bread
⅛ TSP. PEPPER—0

$$\frac{18 \text{ meat}}{8} = 2.25 = 2 \text{ meat}$$

$$\frac{15 \text{ fat}}{8} = 1.88 = 2 \text{ fat}$$

$$\frac{17 \text{ bread}}{8} = 2.13 = 2 \text{ bread}$$

$$\frac{6\frac{1}{2} \text{ veg.}}{8} = 0.8 = 1 \text{ veg.}$$

*8 oz. raw meat is approximately equivalent to 6 oz. cooked meat.

BAKED MACARONI AND CHEESE (SERVES 8)
16 OZ. MACARONI—17.6 BREAD
3 TB. BUTTER—9 FAT
3 TB. FLOUR—1 BREAD
2 C SKIM MILK—2 MILK
SALT AND PEPPER—0
8 OZ. CHEDDAR CHEESE—8 MEAT, 8 FAT
1 C DRY BREAD CRUMBS—2 BREAD

$$\frac{20\frac{1}{2} \text{ BREAD}}{8} = 2.56 = 2\frac{1}{2} \text{ BREAD}$$

$$\frac{17 \text{ FAT}}{8} = 2.13 = 2 \text{ FAT}$$

$$\frac{2 \text{ MILK}}{8} = 0.25 = 0$$

CHICKEN CROQUETTES (SERVES 2)
1 C COOKED, BONED, SKINNED CHICKEN—4 MEAT
1 MED. ONION—1 VEG.
1 GREEN PEPPER—1 VEG.
1 EGG—1 MEAT, ½ FAT
½ C SKIM-MILK BUTTERMILK—½ MILK
SALT AND PEPPER—0

$$\frac{5 \text{ MEAT}}{2} = 2\frac{1}{2} \text{ MEAT}$$

$$\frac{2 \text{ VEG.}}{2} = 1 \text{ VEG.}$$

Let us use the recipe for "chow mein" in a 1000-calorie meal plan and then in a 1500-calorie meal plan.

1000 CALORIE, PLAN B

TOTAL EXCHANGES: 2 MILK, 5 MEAT, 3 FAT, 4 BREAD, 3 FRUIT, 2 VEG.
BREAKFAST: 1 MILK, 1 MEAT, 1 BREAD, 1 FRUIT, ½ FAT
LUNCH: 2 MEAT, 1 BREAD, 1 FRUIT, 1 VEG., ½ FAT
DINNER: 1 MILK, 2 MEAT, 2 FAT, 2 BREAD, 1 FRUIT, 1 VEG.

Breakfast	Lunch	Dinner
8 OZ. SKIM MILK—1 MILK	½ C COTTAGE CHEESE—2 MEAT	1 SERVING CHOW MEIN—2 MEAT,
1 EGG—1 MEAT, ½ FAT	½ C PINEAPPLE—1 FRUIT	2 FAT, 2 BREAD, 1 VEG.
½ C MASHED POTATOES—1	3 RYE WAFERS—1 BREAD	8 OZ. SKIM MILK—1 MILK
BREAD	VEG. PLATE—1 VEG.	½ C PEACHES—1 FRUIT
1 TANGERINE—1 FRUIT	1 TB. VEG. DIP—½ FAT	

1500 CALORIE

TOTAL EXCHANGES: 2 MILK, 5 MEAT, 6 FAT, 8 BREAD, 4 FRUIT, 3 VEG.
BREAKFAST: 1 MILK, 1 MEAT, 2 FAT, 2 BREAD, 1 FRUIT
LUNCH: 2 MEAT, 1 FAT, 4 BREAD, 2 FRUIT, 1 VEG.
DINNER: 1 MILK, 2 MEAT, 3 FAT, 2 BREAD, 1 FRUIT, 2 VEG.

Breakfast	Lunch	Dinner
8 OZ. SKIM MILK—1 MILK	½ C TUNA—2	1 SERVING CHOW MEIN—2 MEAT,
1 EGG—1 MEAT, ½ FAT	2 SL. WW BREAD—2 BREAD	2 FAT, 2 BREAD, 1 VEG.
1 MUFFIN—1 BREAD	1 TSP. MAYONNAISE—1 FAT	1 C TOSSED SALAD—1 VEG.
½ TSP. BUTTER—½ FAT	CELERY, PEPPERS—1 VEG.	1 TB. SALAD DRESSING—1 FAT
½ C FRIED POTATOES—	2 EARS CORN-ON-COB—2 BREAD	8 OZ. SKIM MILK—1 MILK
1 BREAD, 1 FAT	1 LARGE APPLE—2 FRUIT	¼ SM. CANTALOUPE—1 FRUIT
½ C ORANGE JUICE—1 FRUIT		

CHAPTER 10

Getting There Faster

After you have been on a walking program for four weeks, you are ready to begin a serious exercise program. A program designed for you is known as an exercise prescription. However, before you begin any exercise that is more strenuous than walking, we recommend that you have a complete medical checkup. If you are over thirty, it is recommended that the medical checkup include a stress EKG.

Aerobic Activity

There are three types of exercises: cardiovascular endurance, flexibility, and muscular endurance. If your goal is to increase your cardiovascular endurance, the exercise may be any that involves large muscle masses and is performed continuously for a significant period of time. This kind of exercise is known as *aerobic*. Walking is an excellent aerobic exercise, if done briskly for a long enough time. Other aerobic exercises include running, jogging, swimming, cycling, trampolining, cross-country skiing, skating, rope jumping, and dancercise. (Dancercise consists of a series of fifteen to twenty minutes of continuous calisthenics performed with accompanying dance music.)

To build up your cardiovascular system it is necessary that your physical activity be of sufficient intensity and duration to reach what is known as your "training level." This is the level at which your heart muscles will be strengthened to be able to pump more blood per beat, your circulatory system will expand to carry more blood, and your muscles will respond to the additional oxygen and nutrients by manufacturing more muscle tissue, more fuel-burning enzymes, and more mitochondria powerhouses.

Your heart rate during participation in an activity is a fairly reliable measure of the intensity of that participation. There is a maximum rate above which you cannot push your heart. It has been found that this maximum heart rate is dependent upon age, and is independent of other factors. Men and women of the same age have nearly the same maximum heart rates; athletes and sedentary persons of the same age have the same maximum heart rate. The heart will not beat any faster. Research has shown that a training effect occurs when your heart beats at 70 to 80 percent of your predicted maximum heart rate. Figure 12, given below, shows the 70 percent and the 80 percent heart rate for persons of various ages. It is recommended that when you begin an exercise program, you start at your 70 percent training rate and gradually over a period of several weeks work up to your 80 percent rate. If you have a history of heart disease, you should not exceed the 75 percent heart rate.

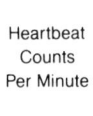
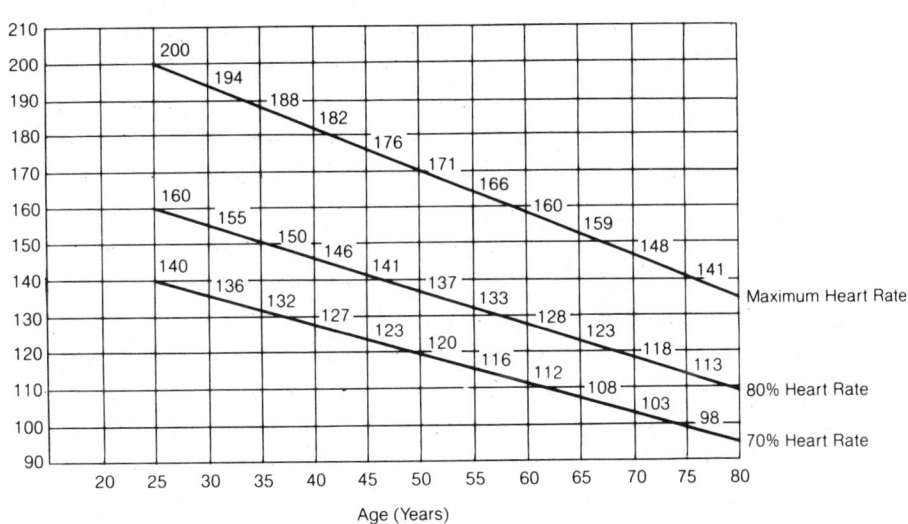

Fig. 12   Maximum Heart Rate and 70% and 80% Level for Various Ages

If you are very sedentary or very much overweight, you might wonder if you should start out at your 70 percent heart rate. Definitely, yes. But do realize that a slow walk might be the 70 percent heart rate for you. This is why it is so important that you monitor your heart rate—so you won't overexert yourself. Perhaps when you begin a walking program, a slow walk will raise your heart rate to the 70 percent level. But as you keep up the program, you will gradually have to increase your speed to maintain that 70 percent level. By this you will know that your physical condition is improving.

To find out if you are performing an activity—walking, running, jogging, cycling, etc.—at your training level, follow this procedure: Perform the activity for two or three minutes at a pace where you experience mild breathlessness, but you are still able to carry on a conversation. Stop. Immediately take your pulse at your wrist or neck. (Practice taking your resting pulse several times before you begin the activity; your pulse will be harder to find when your heart is beating rapidly.) Count your pulse for exactly ten seconds immediately after you stop the activity; then multiply that count by six to obtain your heart rate in beats per minute. (It is suggested that you take your pulse for ten seconds rather than the fifteen to thirty seconds used by medical professionals, because your pulse rate slows down very rapidly after you stop exercising.)

To make the procedure simpler, below is given the ten-second rate for the 70 percent and 80 percent training levels for various ages. All you need to do is to memorize the ten-second heart rate for your age. Then when you are walking, jogging, cycling, etc., stop every so often to check your heart rate.

TABLE 11 TEN–SECOND HEART RATE

AGE	70% RATE	80% RATE	AGE	70% RATE	80% RATE
25	23	27	50	20	23
30	23	26	55	19	22
35	22	25	60	19	21
40	21	24	65	18	21
45	21	24	70	17	20
			75	16	19
			80	16	18

It is very important that your aerobic activity be preceded by a five-minute warm-up and followed by a five-minute cool-down period. It is simplest to begin with five minutes of a slower version of the activity, then perform the activity at your training rate for twenty minutes, then conclude with five minutes of the slower version. Your pulse should be down below one hundred beats per minute (sixteen beats per ten seconds) before you completely stop the activity.

One basic rule is to avoid overexertion at any time. Signs of overexertion are tightness or pain in your chest, severe breathlessness, light-headedness, dizziness, loss of muscle control, and nausea. If you experience any of these symptoms, stop exercising immediately.

ASSIGNMENT 6. *Aerobic Exercise:*

With your partners, if possible, select some aerobic activities that you are all willing and able to participate in. One of the best aerobic activities is walking —just continue your walking program, but now make sure you are walking at your 70 percent training level. (It is important to have partners with similar

NAME _Jennie_

DATE	ACTIVITY	TIME STARTED	TIME ENDED	TEN-SECOND PULSE RATE
6/6	walking	6:35	6:55	21
6/7	walking	6:35	6:55	21
6/8	walking	6:35	6:55	21
6/9	walking	6:35	6:55	21
6/10	walking	6:35	6:55	21
6/11	walking	9:30	9:50	21
6/12				
6/13	walking	6:35	6:55	21
6/14	walking	6:35	6:55	21
6/15	walking	6:35	6:55	21
6/16	walking	6:35	6:55	21
6/17	walking	6:35	6:55	21
6/18	walking	6:35	6:55	21
6/19				
6/20	walking	6:40	7:00	21
6/21	Tennis	6:30	7:30	
6/22	Walking	6:35	6:55	21
6/23	Tennis	6:30	7:30	
6/24	walking	6:40	7:00	21
6/25	walking	6:35	6:55	21
6/26				
6/27	walking	6:35	6:55	21
6/28	Tennis	6:30	7:30	
6/29	walking	6:35	6:55	21
6/30	Tennis	6:30	7:30	
7/1	walking	6:35	6:55	21
7/2	walking	9:40	10:00	21
7-3				
7/4	walking	6:35	6:55	21
7/5	walking	6:30	6:50	21
7/6	walking	6:35	6:55	21
7/7	racquetball	6:30	7:30	
7/8	walking	6:35	6:55	21
7/9	walking	9:35	9:55	21
7/10				
7/11	walking	6:35	6:55	21
7/12	walking	6:35	6:55	21
7/13	tennis	6:30	7:30	
7/14	walking	6:35	6:55	21

GETTING THERE FASTER

training rates.) Begin with five minutes of some warm-up activities; then perform your selected aerobic activity for twenty minutes without stopping. Follow the aerobic activity with five minutes of cool-down activities. Follow this program for five days a week, if possible, but at least for every other day. Continue for six weeks. Keep a record of your performance on Worksheet #6. (A sample worksheet is shown on p. 103; blank worksheets are found in Appendix C.)

The good feeling you have each time you finish the aerobic activity will probably be sufficient reward. However, you might plan some very nice reward —such as new jogging shoes or a new swimsuit or slacks—to be obtained at the end of the six weeks.

Toning Exercises

Exercises that increase flexibility and muscular strength and endurance we shall call "toning" exercises. Flexibility exercises, which consist of slow sustained stretching, help prevent much of muscle soreness. Calisthenics can be used effectively to improve muscle endurance and strength when repeated frequently and regularly.

Toning Exercises

These exercises are designed to (1) strengthen muscle groups, and (2) increase flexibility, and should be done every day.

Deep Knee Bend:

Beginners should hold onto a chair with one hand for balance. Lower yourself into the full squat position, then return to standing position. Keep your head up, your back flat. Do not bounce. Beginners may perform this exercise on their toes. As you progress and can maintain balance, perform this exercise flat-footed. Repeat 10 times.

This exercise strengthens the thighs, buttocks, and lower back; promotes flexibility in the knees and ankles.

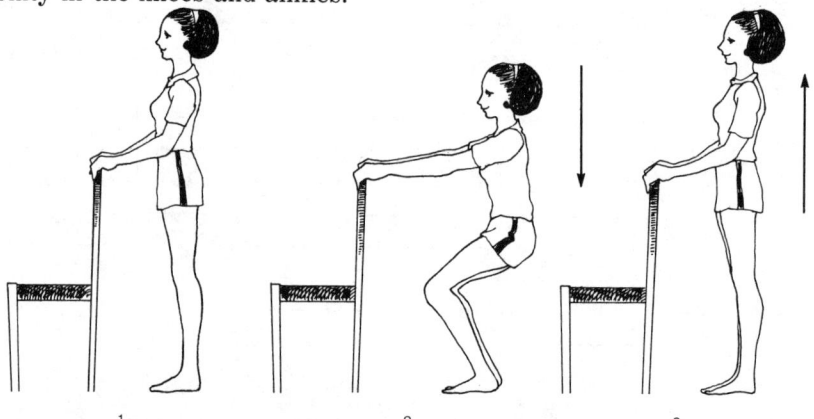

1   2   3

Standing Twist:

Stand, extend arms outward horizontally, and twist the upper body and arms 90 degrees to the right; return to original position. Repeat twisting to the left. Repeat 10 times each side.

This exercise promotes a high degree of flexibility in the torso and the entire abdominal area.

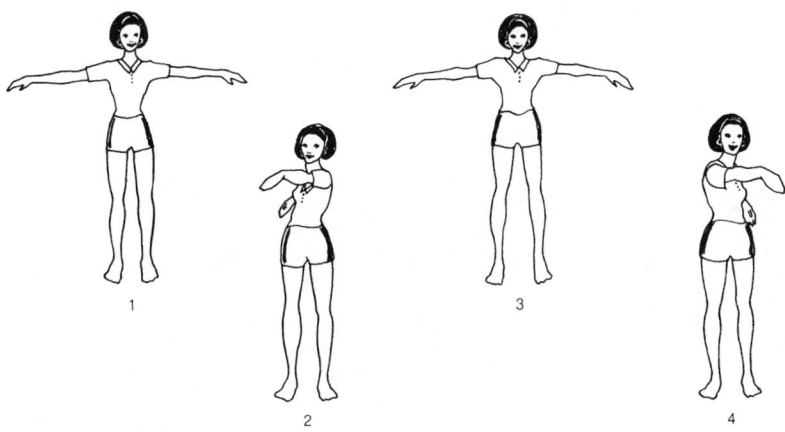

Push-off Wall:

Stand facing a wall and far enough back that your palms can just reach flat against the wall when you fall forward. Slowly allow your upper body to come as close as possible to contact with the wall. Then push back to your original position. Repeat complete sequence 10 times; no halfway repetition.

This exercise strengthens and tones upper body muscles.

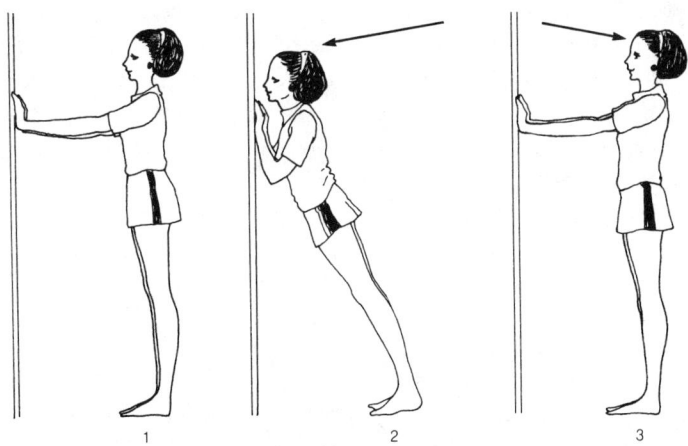

Leg-over:

Lie on your back with your arms extended to the sides at shoulder level. Raise your left leg to a vertical position, keeping your legs straight. Twist your body to touch your left leg to your right hand. Hold 3–5 seconds. Return to starting position. Repeat to the opposite side. Repeat 5 times to each side.

This exercise strengthens and stretches the trunk rotator muscles.

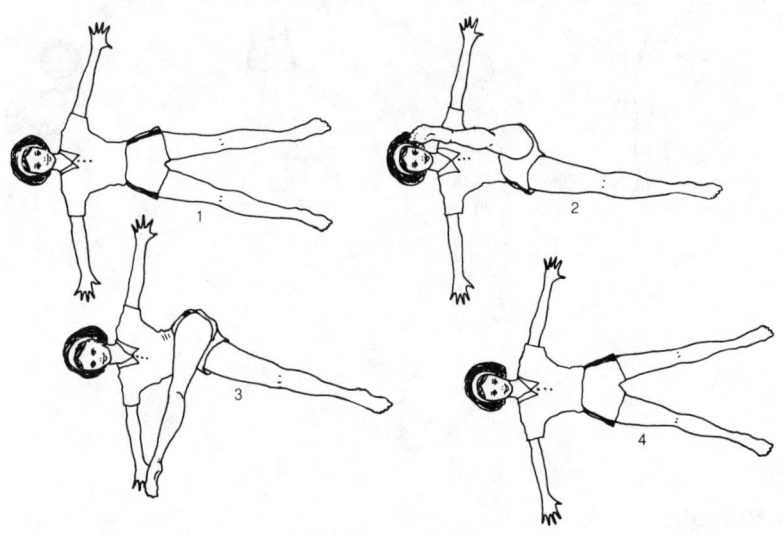

ASSIGNMENT #7. *Toning Exercises:*

Perform the above toning exercises every day for six weeks. Ideally these exercises should be performed during the same six weeks as your aerobic exercises. Keep a record of your performance on Worksheet #7. (A sample worksheet is given on p. 108; blank worksheets are found in Appendix C.)

Since for most people toning exercises are a "chore," you will probably need to plan for a reward to give yourself each week. At the end of six weeks of success give yourself a nice reward.

Extra-Fuel Foods

In planning your meals include all the exchanges of each food group that are allowed on the basic diet. Let us reemphasize: Never, never substitute sugar or alcohol exchanges, or extra-fuel foods, for any food on the basic diet. But, you say, "Couldn't I just substitute those chocolate-chip cookies for the bread or cereal in the basic diet; it's the same number of calories?" The answer is no. The object of the meal planning is not just to obtain a diet with 1000 or 1500 calories —you could do this with straight sugar. The objective is to have a nutritionally balanced diet with a reduced number of calories. While you are trying to lose weight, it is best that you do not eat any extra-fuel foods. However there will probably be times when you *must* have some sweets, or a Coke, or a beer. That is okay as long as you are willing to pay the price. The price is simply that you increase your physical activity enough to "burn up" the extra calories in the extra-fuel foods (increased activity over what you normally expend with your aerobic activity program). Table 13 in Appendix B gives the calorie content of some extra-fuel foods; Tables 14 and 15 give the calorie expenditure of several activities. To determine the "price" of a certain extra-fuel food you merely determine how long you would have to engage in a certain activity to burn up the fuel from the food. Are you willing to pay the price? Decide *before* you eat the food.

Let us take an example to show you how to pay the price. Say for dessert you have four chocolate-chip cookies, which contain about 200 calories. To burn up those extra calories you can walk for about sixty-six minutes (depending on your weight), or cycle for forty minutes, or play a vigorous game of table tennis for fifty minutes. You may select any activity that you wish. The important thing is for you to burn up the extra fuel the same day that you ate the food. Then you do not have to worry about storing the extra calories as fat.

Paying the price with a physical activity is a very easy (and hard) way to account for extra-fuel foods. Also, you achieve a triple bonus by using this method: (1) You will use up the extra calories in physical activity rather than storing them as fat, (2) the activity will make your body feel better, and (3) the extra activity will reduce your desire for more extra-fuel food.

ASSIGNMENT #8. *Extra-Fuel Foods:*
On Worksheet #8 list all of your extra-fuel foods as you eat them; then list the activities that you used to burn up the extra fuel. (A sample worksheet is given on p. 109; blank worksheets are found in Appendix C.)

DATE	EXERCISE	MINS.	DATE	EXERCISE	MINS.
6/6	DKB, ST, POW, LO		6/29	DKB, ST, POW, LO	
6/7	''		6/30	''	
6/8	''		7/1	''	
6/9	''		7/2	''	
6/10	''		7/3	''	
6/11	''		7/4	''	
6/13	''		7/5	''	
6/14	''		7/6	''	
6/15	''		7/7	''	
6/16	''		7/8	''	
6/17	''		7/9	''	
6/18	''		7/11	''	
6/20	''		7/12	''	
6/21	''		7/13	''	
6/22	''		7/14	''	
6/23	''		7/15	''	
6/24	''		7/16	''	
6/25	''		7/18	''	
6/27	''		7/19	''	
6/28	''		7/20	''	

REWARDS: STATE DATE AND TYPE OF REWARD

6/11 – A new book	6/25 – Go to the ballet
6/18 A movie	7/2 Attend a play

NAME Jennie   WEEK OF May 12-18

Date Time	Place	Food and Amount	Calories	Energy Equivalent	E. F. Price Paid Time
Tues 4 PM	Kitchen	4 chocolate chip cookies	200	60 min walk	walked 7 - 8 PM
Fri 4 PM	snack bar	1 12 oz. Coke	145	$\frac{145}{5.2} = 28$ min. walk	walked 7 - 7:30 PM

CHAPTER 11

Avoiding the Potholes

Introduction

You may find that after you increase your physical activity and balance your diet, you do not have any more eating problems. However, you may find that you still have a tendency to eat when you are not hungry. If so this chapter is for you. But first you need to find out your particular problems.

ASSIGNMENT #9. *Analysis of the Food and Behavior Record:*
We asked you to keep a "food and behavior" record when you began this program (see p. 72). Now we want you to complete another "food and behavior" record for an additional week so you can compare the two weeks and determine your progress so far. After you fill out the record form for the second week, complete the data analysis chart, Worksheet #9, for each of the two weeks. (Blank worksheets are given in Appendix C.) After you have completed the data analysis worksheet, determine your behavior problems using the criteria given below:

There are three types of problems that we will consider: (1) external stimuli, (2) quantity of food intake, and (3) mood eating.

WORKSHEET #9. ANALYSIS OF FOOD-AND-BEHAVIOR RECORD

HOW MANY TIMES EACH DAY DID YOU:	SUN Week 1	SUN Week 2	MON Week 1	MON Week 2	TUE Week 1	TUE Week 2	WED Week 1	WED Week 2	THU Week 1	THU Week 2	FRI Week 1	FRI Week 2	SAT Week 1	SAT Week 2	TOTAL Week 1	TOTAL Week 2
1. Eat something?	7	6	9	6	10	8	9	7	10	7	9	6	10	7	64	47
2. Eat empty-calorie foods?	7	1	8	0	7	1	7	1	8	1	8	0	8	1	52	5
3. Eat not sitting at a table?	5	3	6	2	7	3	5	2	6	2	6	3	7	4	42	19
4. Eat while doing other things?	5	3	7	3	7	2	4	2	7	2	6	3	7	4	43	19
5. Eat alone at nonmealtimes?	0	0	1	0	5	2	2	2	4	1	2	3	5	0	19	8
6. Eat with a friend at nonmealtimes?	5	3	5	0	3	0	4	0	4	0	4	0	3	4	28	7
7. Eat when you were feeling bored?	2	0	1	2	1	2	0	0	3	0	2	0	1	0	10	4
8. Eat when feeling restless?	3	0	0	0	2	1	2	1	3	1	2	2	2	2	14	8
9. Eat when feeling angry or unhappy?	0	0	0	0	0	1	2	0	0	0	1	0	2	0	5	4
10. Eat when feeling worried?	0	0	0	0	0	2	0	1	1	0	0	0	2	0	3	3
11. Eat when feeling lonely?	0	0	0	0	0	0	0	0	0	0	0	0	0	0	0	0
12. Gorge yourself with one certain food?	0	0	0	0	0	0	0	0	0	0	0	0	0	0	0	0
13. Eat large amounts of food?	6	0	0	0	0	0	0	0	0	0	0	0	0	0	0	0
14. Eat when you were not hungry?	5	0	6	2	8	2	8	2	4	1	6	0	7	1	44	8

Controlling External Stimuli

External stimuli problems are indicated by:

1. Eating more often than three or six times a day.
2. Eating in rooms other than a normal meal room.
3. Eating not sitting at a table.
4. Eating while watching TV, reading, or performing other activities.
5. Eating always with a certain person—or alone—at nonmealtimes.
6. Eating when not hungry.

You can overcome these problems by rearranging your environment and controlling your external stimuli in the following ways:

1. Eliminate the presence of food—"fat-proof" your house.
   A. Keep food out of sight by:
      1. Removing all dishes of candy, nuts, chips, etc., from your rooms.
      2. Not leaving cakes, cookies, or pies sitting on the kitchen counters.
      3. Placing snack foods in a covered container at the back of a shelf.
      4. Putting snack foods into the refrigerator.
      5. Cleaning up leftovers immediately after a meal.

   B. Avoid buying extra-fuel snack foods:
      1. Shop on a full stomach; you are much more likely to buy on impulse when you are hungry.
      2. Make a shopping list before going to the market; then buy only the items on the list.
      3. Shop alone. Do not take anyone who will urge you to buy snack foods. If you have small children, you might arrange baby-sitting exchanges with a friend to enable you to shop alone.
      4. Shop only the aisles that contain the foods you are intending to buy. Do not even walk down problem food aisles.

2. Break the association between food and other activities.
   A. Eat only while sitting down at the table in an appropriate meal room.
   B. Make eating a "pure experience."
      1. Enjoy your food without distractions.
      2. Carry on a conversation with your associates, but do nothing else except eat.
   C. Make eating a very special experience: Every time you eat *anything*

(even a cookie or an apple), set a plate, glass, utensils, napkin, and place mat.

ASSIGNMENT #10. *Controlling External Stimuli:*
Practice the principles of behavior modification to help you change your habitual way of responding to external stimuli. On the goal-setting chart found in Appendix C, list your goals, your environmental changes, and your practices to help you control external stimuli. Record your success and rewards. Extend your goals. You may use the suggestions given here or other suggestions you have heard. A sample goal-setting chart is shown on p. 114.

Controlling the Amount of Food Intake

Food quantity problems are indicated by:

1. Eating large amounts of food at meals.
2. Eating large amounts of food between meals.
3. Gorging yourself with food at any time.

Suggestions for rearranging your environment and practices to help you control the amount of food that you eat are the following:

1. Eat your food slowly:
    A. Take small bites—not huge mouthfuls. Take small sips of a liquid.
    B. Chew your food thoroughly. Perhaps chew twenty times before swallowing.
    C. Set down your eating utensils between bites.

2. Take small portions:
    A. Use the smallest container possible. (A small amount of food is psychologically more satisfying if it completely fills the container.)
    B. Keep the serving dishes off the table during the meal. (The temptation for seconds is less if food is out of sight and reach.)
    C. Cook only enough food for one serving for each person eating. (Thus no leftovers available for snacking.)

ASSIGNMENT #11. *Controlling Food Intake Amount:*
On a goal-setting chart found in Appendix C, list your goals, your environmental changes, and your practices to help you control your food intake amounts. Record your successes and rewards. Extend your goals. A sample goal-setting chart is shown on p. 115.

10 September   GOAL-SETTING CHART

MY GOALS WILL BE:

1. Eat only at mealtimes for one week.

2.

3.

I WILL REARRANGE MY ENVIRONMENT BY:

1. "Fat-proof" my house.

2.

3.

I WILL PRACTICE:

	M	T	W	T	F	S	S
1. Keep all food out of sight between meals	✓	✓	✓	✓	✓	✓	✓
2. Not buy extra fuel foods	✓	✓	✓	✓	✓		✓
3. Eat only while sitting at table in dining room (or lunch room)	✓		✓	✓			✓
4. Not read or watch TV while eating	✓	✓			✓		
5. Eat only at mealtimes	✓		✓	✓	✓		

I WILL REWARD MYSELF FOR SUCCESS BY:

1. For every 10 checkmarks, I will buy myself a new record

2.

3.

I WILL EXTEND MY GOAL:

	M	T	W	T	F	S	S	M	T	W	T	F	S	S
1.	✓	✓	✓	✓	✓	✓	✓	✓	✓	✓	✓	✓	✓	✓
2.	✓	✓		✓	✓	✓	✓	✓	✓	✓	✓	✓	✓	✓
3.	✓	✓			✓		✓		✓	✓	✓		✓	✓
4.	✓	✓	✓			✓	✓	✓		✓	✓	✓	✓	✓
5.	✓		✓	✓		✓		✓		✓		✓	✓	✓

Controlling Mood Eating Problems

Mood eating problems are indicated by:

1. Nonmeal eating when you are feeling bored, unhappy, restless, angry, worried, or lonely.
2. Eating when not hungry.
3. Eating many empty-calorie or extra-fuel foods.
4. Eating alone at nonmeal times.

After you recognize that you have a problem with mood eating and set a goal to overcome the problem, the most successful way to rearrange your environment is to be prepared. Be prepared with activities to substitute for eating when the problem emotion strikes. (You need to be prepared beforehand because often while you are experiencing the problem emotion, you are not able to think of any substitute activity.) If you have prepared several substitute activities to be used "in case of emergency," whenever the problem emotion arises, you can substitute one of the planned alternative activities for eating. Eventually you will establish the habit of performing the substitute activity whenever you experience the problem emotion. Thus you will break the association between the emotion and eating. In the process you will establish some beneficial associations between the emotion and various activities.

ASSIGNMENT #12. *Substitute Activities for Mood Eating:*
Fill out Worksheet #12, Controlling Moods, found in Appendix C. First list possible activities that you could substitute for eating. List some pleasant nonessential activities such as going to a movie or window shopping, and some essential activities like washing windows or the car. Then list situations that might

occur in your life that are apt to be accompanied by a problem emotion. List the expected situation and then list a specific activity that you will engage in while you are experiencing the problem emotion.

On the last part of the worksheet record each situation that brings on a problem emotion as it happens. Give yourself a reward each time you were able to substitute a nonfood activity for mood eating. A sample worksheet is shown below.

WORKSHEET 12   CONTROLLING MOODS WITH SUBSTITUTE ACTIVITIES

SUBSTITUTE ACTIVITIES:
PLEASANT ACTIVITIES

Walking   Visiting friends

Reading   Taking a class

Sewing   Buying a book

Painting   Seeing a movie

Playing with dog   Window shopping

NECESSARY ACTIVITIES:

Working

House cleaning

Household repairs

Car repair

SITUATIONS WHERE ACTIVITY WILL BE USED:

1. When I get angry with Bob, go for a walk
2. When I'm bored, do housework
3. When I'm tense, visit or call a friend
4. When I have the blues, take the dog to the park
5. When I'm restless, do some painting
6.
7.
8.
9.
10.
11.
12.
13.
14.
15.

SITUATIONS WHEN ACTIVITY WAS ACTUALLY USED:

1. March 25 - Bored - dusted all the books
2. March 28 - Angry with Bob - went for a walk
3. March 29 - Tense, worried - visited Elizabeth

AVOIDING THE POTHOLES

4. <u>April 5 - Restless - started sketch for new painting</u>

5. <u>April 7 - The blues - walked in the park with Thunder</u>

6. _____

7. _____

8. _____

9. _____

10. _____

CHAPTER 12

Moving On

Perhaps the least discussed and most often failed part of any weight-control program is that of sustaining your optimal weight. If you have succeeded in the program to this point, then it really should be something like coasting. There are two main ingredients: an activity program and a maintenance diet. The activity program will consist of nothing more than continuing the toning and aerobic exercises that you have found so fulfilling. The maintenance diet permits more calories per day than the weight-loss diet and includes a wider variety of exchanges. After it is used for a few months, it will evolve into a pattern that includes most of your old favorites, but in smaller amounts. Welcome, then, to the new, *permanently changed* you!

Planning Your Own Lifelong Activity Program

When you write your exercise prescription, you decide what type of exercise you will perform, and for how long you will perform it. To be of real value, your activity program must be one that you will continue for the rest of your life. Since cardiovascular endurance is the most important component of overall fitness, let us first consider the principles involved in designing an aerobic activity program.

1. *Type of activity.* Your cardiovascular system will be improved most effectively by exercises that involve the large muscle groups of the hips and legs, that are rhythmic, and that are continuous for at least twenty minutes. Some suitable activities are walking, jogging, running, cycling, swimming, cross-country skiing, rope jumping, and dancing.

However, perhaps you have a problem with your feet or legs that makes it impossible to be on your feet very much. For you a stationary bicycle might provide the best exercise. Maybe you are embarrassed to go outside where other people can watch you. For you dancercise or a mini-trampoline exercise might be best.

2. *Intensity.* To develop your cardiovascular system, the intensity of your activity must be great enough to work your heart and develop your heart muscles. To accomplish this you need to perform the activity at your 70 percent or 80 percent training level. However, you should not go over your 80 percent training level unless you are a trained athlete. (If the intensity is too great for you, the activity will be anaerobic, rather than aerobic; this will lead to rapid fatigue and perhaps some tissue damage. In addition you will be burning glucose, rather than the fatty acids that you are trying to get out of your adipose cell storage.) Most beginners start out too fast. Slow down; your best improvement will be when your heart is working at 70 percent to 80 percent of its maximum capacity. Also, at that rate you will find the activity enjoyable.

3. *Duration.* To be of value to your cardiovascular system, you must perform the activity continuously for about twenty minutes. The problem with stop-and-go activities such as tennis, basketball, volleyball, and many other games is that the duration of continuous activity is too short. If you perform the activity for only five or ten minutes, regardless of the intensity, it doesn't help your heart. It is much more helpful to walk for twenty minutes than to run for five minutes. If you perform the activity at *your* training rate, you can easily keep it up for twenty minutes.

4. *Frequency.* This is the greatest problem for most people; it is so easy to find excuses for "not this time." To develop and maintain your cardiovascular fitness, you must perform the activity at least every other day, week after week. If you take a few days off, your fitness will drop; if you take a few weeks off, you will be back where you started from when you began the program. This is why it is important to select something you enjoy, that is convenient—so you will continue with the activity for the rest of your life.

The toning exercises have been found to be effective for a reasonable level of fitness. However, you might wish to combine calisthenics with some weight training. If so, that is the kind of exercise that you plan. The particular program you select should be something that you like to do and, hence, something that you can work into your own life-style.

We recommend a minimum of twenty minutes of aerobic activity plus five minutes of toning exercises. In designing aerobic activities, plan for inclement weather and emergencies. If the weather is too wet for walking, what will you do instead? Jump rope? Dancercise? Run up and down stairs? How will you work around the invariable emergencies? Get up twenty minutes earlier or go to bed twenty minutes later? Give your exercise program the highest priority. (You might as well, because if your health deteriorates, you won't be able to do these other important things anyway.)

ASSIGNMENT #13. *Your Own Activity Program:*
Design your own activity program using Worksheet #13. Write your plans in sufficient detail that you will know precisely what you are going to do. (A sample worksheet is shown on p. 122; blank worksheets are found in Appendix C.) Carry out your program for one year. Keep a record on Worksheet #14 for at least six weeks. At the end of the year you will feel so good that you will carry it out for another year . . . and live happily ever after.

Planning Maintenance Diets

After you reach your ideal or desired weight, you can modify the basic exchange diets so that you can maintain that weight for the rest of your life. All that you have learned so far about planning exchange diets can be used in planning a maintenance diet. To plan a maintenance diet, first determine the daily calories you need to maintain your desired weight. Next select an exchange diet from those given on pp. 123–124 with the total number of calories nearest to the value you need for maintenance. Then divide the total exchanges of each food group into three or six meals. All that is left is for you to decide which foods in each group you want to eat each day.

To determine the number of calories you need for your maintenance diet, multiply your desired weight by 13 (for a woman) or 15 (for a man), if your life-style is only moderately active. If you are a very active person, multiply your weight by 15 (for a woman) or 17 (for a man). Table 16 in Appendix B gives approximate desirable weights for men and women. For a more accurate determination, follow the procedure in Table 17, Appendix B.

Let us go through some examples to show you how to determine your daily calories and how to plan your maintenance diets:

EXAMPLE

NANCY'S IDEAL WEIGHT: 140 LBS. MAINTENANCE CALORIES = $140 \times 13 = 1820$

TOTAL EXCHANGES: 2 MILK, 5 MEAT, 8 FAT, 6 FRUIT, 4 VEG., 8 BREAD, 2½ SUGAR
BREAKFAST: 1 MILK, 1 MEAT, ½ FAT, 2 BREAD, 2 FRUIT, ½ SUGAR
LUNCH: 1 MILK, 1 MEAT, 2 FAT, 2 BREAD, 2 FRUIT, 2 VEG., ½ SUGAR
DINNER: 3 MEAT, 5½ FAT, 4 BREAD, 2 FRUIT, 2 VEG., 1½ SUGAR

GOALS:

1. To walk for 20 minutes or more at 80% training rate for 5 or 6 days a week for 52 weeks

2. To perform 20 minutes of toning exercises 5 or 6 days a week for 52 weeks

3. _____

_____

SPECIFIC PLANS:

1. A: To walk or run every day except Sunday.

   B: If weather is too cold or wet — perform 20 minutes of dancercise

   C: If phonograph or radio not available, walk up & down stairs for 20 minutes.

   D: If stairs not available, run in place for 15 minutes.

2. A: To perform toning exercises at beginning and end of day.

B: If oversleep, exercise any way; if late at night, exercise any way.

C: If sick but able to get out of bed – exercise any way.

You will note that sweet desserts can be planned as part of the maintenance diets. Also, if alcoholic beverages are part of your life-style, you can substitute an alcohol exchange for a sugar exchange. For example you can substitute a 12-oz. can of beer (three alcohol exchanges) for three sugar exchanges. However, within the framework of the exchange diet only a limited amount of sugar or alcohol exchanges are permitted each day. If you want more, it is best to treat

MAINTENANCE EXCHANGE DIETS

1800 CALORIE

EXCHANGES	CAL	PRO G	CHO G	FAT G
2 MILK	160	16	24	—
5 MEAT	275	35	—	15
8 FAT	350	—	—	40
8 BREAD	560	16	120	—
6 FRUIT	240	—	60	—
4 VEG.	100	8	20	—
2½ SUGAR	120	—	30	—
TOTAL	1850	75	254	55
%		17	56	27

2000 CALORIE

EXCHANGES	CAL	PRO G	CHO G	FAT G
2½ MILK	200	20	30	—
5½ MEAT	303	39	—	17
9 FAT	405	—	—	45
8 BREAD	560	16	120	—
7 FRUIT	280	—	70	—
4½ VEG.	113	9	23	—
3 SUGAR	144	—	36	—
TOTAL	2005	84	279	62
%		17	56	28

2200 Calorie

2½ MILK	200	20	30	—
6 MEAT	330	42	—	18
10 FAT	450	—	—	50
9 BREAD	630	18	135	—
7 FRUIT	280	—	70	—
5 VEG.	125	10	25	—
4 SUGAR	192	—	48	—
TOTAL	2207	90	308	68
%		16	56	28

2500 Calorie

3 MILK	240	24	36	—
6½ MEAT	358	46	—	20
11½ FAT	518	—	—	58
11 BREAD	770	22	165	—
8 FRUIT	320	—	80	—
5 VEG.	125	10	25	—
4 SUGAR	192	—	48	—
TOTAL	2523	102	354	78
%		16	56	28

2800 Calorie

3 MILK	240	24	36	—
6½ MEAT	358	46	—	20
13 FAT	585	—	—	65
12 BREAD	840	24	180	—
9 FRUIT	360	—	90	—
5½ VEG.	138	11	28	—
6 SUGAR	288	—	72	—
TOTAL	2809	105	406	85
%		15	58	27

3000 Calorie

3 MILK	240	24	36	—
6½ MEAT	358	46	—	20
14 FAT	630	—	—	70
13 BREAD	910	26	195	—
10 FRUIT	400	—	100	—
6 VEG.	150	12	30	—
7 SUGAR	336	—	84	—
TOTAL	3024	108	445	90
%		14	59	27

CALCULATION OF % PROTEIN, CARBOHYDRATE, AND FAT: EACH GRAM OF PROTEIN AND EACH GRAM OF CARBOHYDRATE CONTAIN 4 CALORIES. EACH GRAM OF FAT CONTAINS 9 CALORIES.

75 GRAMS PROTEIN $\times$ 4 CALORIES/GRAM = 300 CALORIES FROM PROTEIN
254 GRAMS CARBOHYDRATE $\times$ 4 CALORIES/GRAM = 1016 CALORIES FROM CARBOHYDRATE
55 GRAMS FAT $\times$ 9 CALORIES/GRAM = 495 CALORIES FROM FAT

$$\frac{300}{1811} = 16.6\% \text{ PROTEIN}; \quad \frac{1016}{1811} = 56.1\% \text{ CARBOHYDRATE}; \quad \frac{495}{1811} = 27.3\% \text{ FAT}$$

the extra exchanges as extra-fuel food and burn off the extra calories with physical activity. It is very important to account for all extra-fuel foods; either as part of the exchange diet or to be burned off with extra physical activity.

You should plan and follow your maintenance diet meals for several weeks. Weigh yourself every day for two weeks; if your weight increases more than two pounds, reduce the number of fat or sugar or alcohol exchanges. Check your weight each day for another two weeks. Continue this adjusting until you have a maintenance exchange diet that is just right for you.

ASSIGNMENT #14. *Maintenance Meal Planning:*
Using the meal-planning forms found in Appendix C, Worksheet #15, plan your meals according to the exchange diet you have selected. Follow your plan for two weeks. If your weight remains constant ($\pm$ 2 lbs.), continue writing down and following your meal plans for another four to eight weeks. If after the first two weeks you find you are gaining weight, decrease your fat or sugar ex-

changes and make a new set of meal plans. Continue making adjustments in the exchange diet until you have one that will maintain your weight. Follow this exchange diet for another four to eight weeks.

Continue your maintenance meal planning until those plans become part of your life-style.

Planning for Prevention

As any overweight person well knows, the best time to begin a weight-control program is *before* you become overweight. It is much easier not to store that extra fat in the first place than it is to try to get rid of the fat after it is stored. The best time to plan for prevention is in childhood, before fat-storing eating and activity habits are well established. Prevention programs are most effective when the entire family is involved.

How can you plan for overweight prevention? Let us consider the Wells family to find out how they succeeded. Mark, a heavy-equipment operator, and Judy, a homemaker, have three children: Lori, age ten; Brent, age eight; and Susan, age four. Mark and Judy both are "somewhat plump." After getting off the scales one evening Mark and Judy decided to begin a weight-control program. They also decided to help their children avoid becoming overweight as teen-agers.

The first thing they decided to do was to increase their physical activity. Judy realized that she spent most of her day in the house, and Mark knew that he spent most of his day in a driver's seat. Judy decided to jog each morning with Lori and Brent, while Mark and Susan prepared breakfast. While the older children were in school, Judy decided to walk with Susan on her tricycle around the neighborhood. Then when Lori and Brent got home from school, they would all walk to the park to play on the playground equipment.

Mark decided that he would run with a friend for thirty minutes of their lunch hours. Then in the evenings Mark would put Susan on his bicycle and they would all ride around the community for an hour. They bought a season's pass to the community swimming pool and planned to go there two evenings a week. They bought some new phonograph records and planned dancercise sessions for bad-weather days.

Mark and Judy also decided to control the food environment in their home. For snacks they provided fresh or dried fruit or some crunchy vegetable. For desserts they had canned fruits or fresh or frozen melons or berries. They planned their meals around the basic exchange diets, making sure that they and their children had adequate numbers of exchanges of each food group. Soon the children began to prefer apples to cookies, oranges to cake. Birthday parties and special holidays were still a problem, but eating plans are not wrecked by a few exceptions.

Judy and Mark had previously had many problems with eating in response to external stimuli. It helped a great deal not to have extra-fuel foods available. Judy's worst time was during the day, so she decided that whenever she craved food, she would get involved in some housework that was not compatible with eating—such as washing dishes or washing windows. Mark's problem was in the evening after the children were in bed. He decided to spend that time in his basement workshop making Christmas toys for the children.

After a year Mark and Judy both had their weight down to normal and they "felt great!" The children loved the extra time their parents spent with them. The whole family approved of their new life-style.

Let us consider some reasons why the Wells family was successful in their weight-control program:

1. Both parents realized that their weight-control program should involve the entire family.
2. The parents taught their children by example to enjoy physical activities and nutritious foods.
3. The physical activities that they selected were "fun." The parents spent time with their children in these activities.
4. The parents learned to substitute other activities for eating in response to external stimuli. They taught this to their children by example.

But suppose your children are teen-agers and don't want to do anything with you? Or your children are grown up and no longer live with you; or you are just married and have no children; or you are single and live alone. How, then, do you plan for prevention? The first thing to realize is that you must begin where you are. The world is full of things undone because of "if only." "If only my parents had raised me differently; If only I had begun earlier; If only my children were younger; If only I were married . . ." Whatever your present situation in life, start there.

If your children are teen-agers, perhaps they would enjoy planning physical activities for the whole family. (Don't expect to keep up with them, though.) Have nutritious snacks readily available at home. And most of all—set the example!

If your children are grown, or you haven't any, plan physical activities with your spouse, or with your spouse and other couples. Work together on meal planning. If you are single, this is a great time to get together with one or more friends to begin activity programs that can develop into lifetime habits. Do you like to cycle? Or go mountain climbing? Or backpacking? Do you like roller skating? Or swimming? You and your friends can plan regular activity times. The important thing is to *do* something! It does not matter if the activities you choose are different from the examples we've provided. It does not matter if the meal plans you design don't match the ones we've discussed. What does matter is that you have an activity plan and a meal plan—and that you follow them.

The whole thrust of this book is to describe basic biological facts about your body in a way that will motivate you to adopt lifelong changes in eating and activity habits. Regardless of whatever motivation comes from this or other sources, the single most important thing for you to do is to decide—right now, today—that you are going to do it. Without that decision this book's principles and plans will only add to the decor of your padded prison of dreams.

Decide, and you open the prison door. Use the book, and you fly free. All it takes is one step at a time. Grab a pen. Fill out Form #1. Do it.

PART III.

Special Energy Needs

Introduction

Often there is a strong urge to adjust one's weight at special times during life. Adolescence is one of these, pregnancy is another. There are special problems and opportunities presented by the substantial changes that occur in bodies during these times of fast tissue growth and hormonal surges. We have prepared these next two chapters as guides for those of you who may be living through one of them now. We urge you to pay great heed to the cautions we cite. No need for weight loss is so urgent as to warrant ignoring the precautions.

CHAPTER 13

Weight Control in Adolescence

As you know, being an overweight teen-ager is no fun. Adolescence is hard enough under the best of circumstances. But when "slim is in" and "fat is out" and you are fat, sometimes life becomes almost unbearable. Is there anything you can do about it? Or are you just destined to be a fatty all your life? The answers to these questions depend very much on you. You now have most of the responsibility for your own body—what you do with it is your own decision. Other teen-agers have been able to reduce the fat stores in their body and to maintain normal weight the rest of their lives. However, it is not easy and you will succeed only if *you* really want to lose that fat.

How much weight do you need to lose? What is your ideal body weight? Some teen-agers approximate a skeleton. However, if you are really overweight, you would probably be happy to lose ten or twenty pounds. To get a rough estimate of your ideal weight, find your height on the proper column in Table 16, Appendix B. Then subtract one pound for each year under twenty-five to get your desirable weight. If you want to determine your ideal weight more accurately, use the procedure given in Table 17, Appendix B.

We want to make one point clear: Losing fat is not necessarily the same as losing weight. We talk about losing weight because that is easy to measure. But what you really want is to lose fat.

Overweight in Adolescence

As an overweight teen-ager you have two problems with your body that adults do not have. One problem is that you are still growing, and you must be very careful to get all the nutrients that your body needs to build new bone and tissue. Crash diets, if carried on very long, are stupid for an adult but are disastrous for a growing teen-ager. If you decide you do not like milk, or that milk is "fattening," you probably won't have enough calcium to build more bone and tissue (and can't grow taller if you don't make more bone tissue). If you do not eat enough high-protein foods, you probably won't have sufficient amino acids to build new tissue for your muscles, skin, heart, and other organs. The right balance of all the nutrients is required for growth of new tissue. In fact, if you do not get the right balance of nutrients, your body can't make new tissue, so it just burns the food you do eat for fuel or stores it as fat.

The first step in planning your weight-control program is to make sure that you have a balance of the nutrients that you need for growth. This is especially important for girls, so you will build up a reserve of the minerals in case you decide at some time to become a mother.

The minimum amount of each of the protective foods for a growing teen-ager are given in the chart below:

FOOD	DAILY AMOUNT
MILK, FORTIFIED WITH VITAMINS A AND D, SKIM OR 2%	4 CUPS
LEAN MEAT, POULTRY, FISH, CHEESE, EGGS	1 EGG DAILY; 4 OZ. MEAT OR CHEESE
BREAD, WHOLE GRAIN	2 SLICES
CEREAL, WHOLE GRAIN	1 CUP
POTATOES, CORN, DRIED BEANS, WINTER SQUASH	¾ CUP
OTHER COOKED VEGETABLES, GREEN OR YELLOW	½ CUP
RAW VEGETABLES	½ CUP
CITRUS FRUITS, TOMATOES, OR PEPPERS	1 LG. ORANGE OR EQUIV.
OTHER FRUITS	2 SERVINGS
UNSATURATED OILS	1 TB

The calories recommended for growing girls and boys are:

	GIRLS	BOYS
11–14 YEARS	25 CAL./LB.	29 CAL./LB.
15–18 YEARS	18 CAL./LB.	22 CAL./LB.

This brings us to the second problem teen-agers have: During your rapid-growth years, the body is able to increase the number of its fat cells. (Before birth, infancy, and adolescence appear to be the three times in life that new adipose cells are manufactured.) Adults, when they get fat, just keep filling up the adipose cells that they already have. But rapidly growing teen-agers can manufacture additional adipose cells. When you make additional cells, it increases the difficulty of losing weight. As we explained in Chapter 1, the adipose cells seem to have a set-point, and your body tries to fill up all the cells to that point. If you have extra adipose cells, your body has to store more fat to fill up all the extra cells.

So how are you going to be able to get all the nutrients you need and yet not manufacture extra adipose cells? First make sure that you consume the minimum amount of protective food listed earlier. After you have done that, then turn your attention to the first principle of a weight-control program:

INCREASE YOUR PHYSICAL ACTIVITY!

Why should you increase your physical activity? First and foremost it will increase your self-esteem. If you have been overweight most of your life, your ego has probably been battered with comments such as, "Fatty can't run," or "Why can't you stick to a diet?" or "Girls don't like fat boys," or "If you weren't so lazy, you wouldn't be so heavy," or "All you ever do is eat and watch TV," or "She can't play ball, she's too fat." By now you may have a pretty poor self-image. You might have concluded that you are a failure—at everything. There are few things so ego-building as the realization that you are able to maintain an exercise program. You can think, "Well, I might not be a good ball player, but I can ride my bike an hour a day, or four miles every day for two months!" You realize that you *do* have willpower. You realize that your body can do something: "I walked two miles every day for four weeks." "I can succeed at something."

In addition to the realization that you can succeed, regular exercise gives your brain another boost. This is sometimes called the "runner's high." People who exercise vigorously and regularly feel a "high" that is better than anything you can get from drugs. It is believed that exercise causes your brain to produce molecules called endorphins, which interact with brain receptors in such a way as to give you a feeling of well-being. This feeling of well-being raises your ego. "I'm okay—all is well with me."

If exercise did nothing more than increase your self-esteem, that would be enough. But there are other benefits: One is that physical activity uses up calories—from your food, if available; otherwise, from your fat stores. Granted, increasing your physical activity does not use up a lot of calories. Riding your bicycle for twenty-five minutes might cause you to use up only 100 calories (the amount in a large apple). But if you bicycle every day for a month, you will use up about 3000 calories, and that is almost equivalent to a pound of fat. And if you bicycle every day for a year, you will use up about 36,000 calories, which is equivalent to about ten pounds of fat. So, just think, you don't have to change anything else except to bicycle every day for twenty-five minutes more than you do now to lose ten pounds in a year.

Another benefit is that regular exercise will cause you to replace fat tissue with muscle tissue. This will make you look slimmer even if you stay the same weight. (Young girls sometimes worry about developing unsightly bulging muscles if they exercise. You don't need to worry about that; your sex hormones and skeletal structure, not exercise, determine your masculinity or femininity.) In addition to looking better, you will use up more calories or energy, even while you are resting, because muscle requires a significant amount of energy just to maintain tone; fat tissue requires hardly any energy at all.

Another benefit that might surprise you is that you will have a decreased desire to eat. You probably know that you eat much of your food when you aren't even hungry. Regular exercise has been found to decrease a person's desire to eat excessively. Regular exercise helps your body realize when it has had enough food; regular exercise helps to prevent you from overeating.

And still more benefits: Regular exercise helps you to have more "energy." If you are overweight, you probably "drag" through the day. You just don't seem to have enough energy to walk to your friend's house, so you stay home and watch TV. Just watch the increase in energy that you will have after a few weeks of regular physical activity.

Now, if you need any more benefits, there is one that will naturally result, but which you probably won't worry about for another twenty years or so. You will have better health. Your chances for such things as a heart attack and diabetic blindness will be reduced. At age fifteen those things are no concern; but there is a good likelihood that someday you will attain age thirty-five or forty-five—and then it will matter.

How do you start a physical activity program? First read the section in Chapters 4 and 10 on aerobic exercises. We recommend that if it is possible, you join some organized group that has regular practices. Children who are overweight during their growing years usually develop stronger-than-normal muscles to cope with the extra weight. Hence an overweight teen-ager has the potential of being very good in sports. Swimming is an excellent sport to begin with, since overweight is not as much a handicap as in something like basketball. If you can swim, and a swim team or an aquatic team is available, we recommend that you join it. Other suggestions of organized activities include bike hiking groups, hiking clubs, karate clubs, tennis teams or classes, dance teams or dance classes. To be useful as an aerobic activity, practices should be at least three times a week.

If you cannot join a class or a team, we recommend that you find a friend or a brother or sister who will join with you in regular physical activity. Select any activity that uses large muscles, such as walking, running, bicycling, that you can perform at least every other day. The activity will probably be hard at first, so take it slowly. However after about six weeks you will be "hooked" on it; then when you miss a day, you will feel something is wrong.

After you are successful in maintaining an activity program for a few weeks, you are ready to tackle dietary restrictions. Realizing that you have the motivation and willpower to continue with a physical activity program helps you to know that you can also manage dietary restrictions. If you are still in your growth spurt, the restrictions do not have to be great because of the large amount of energy that your body needs. Often just a few substitutions are all that is needed. In the chart below are listed some substitutions that will decrease the number of calories you eat and increase the nutritive value of the food. You might at first just make these substitutions.

Original Food	CAL	Significant Nutrients	Substituted Food	CAL	Significant Nutrients
1 C sugared popcorn	134	FIBER	1 C plain popcorn	23	FIBER
3 oz. candy bar	450	0	2 dried apricots	40	IRON, VIT. A
8 oz. milkshake	350	CALCIUM	8 oz. 2% milk	80	CALCIUM, VIT. A, D
1 pc. chocolate cake	365	0	1 pc. melon	40	VIT. C, FIBER
1 brownie	97	0	5 carrot sticks	25	VIT. A, FIBER
3 oatmeal cookies	177	0	1 large apple	80	FIBER, VIT. A, C
1 pc. cherry pie	412	0	1 C cherries	80	FIBER, VIT. A, C
1 raised doughnut	176	0	1 tangerine	40	FIBER, VIT. C
12 oz. coke	144	0	1 C pineapple juice	80	VIT. C
1 Big Mac	550	PROTEIN	1 plain hamburger	260	PROTEIN
2 pc. crispy chicken	665	PROTEIN	2 pc. chicken with skin removed	325	PROTEIN
1 sl. bread and jelly and peanut butter	263	PROTEIN, VIT. B	1 sl. cheddar cheese	100	PROTEIN, CALCIUM

Let's consider a typical day's snacks to see how you can drastically reduce your calorie intake with just a few changes. Perhaps your pattern is to eat a candy bar between your classes at school. After school, you stop at a snack bar for a Coke and a doughnut. When you get home, you have a piece of bread with peanut butter and jelly. You have a piece of cake for your bedtime snack. For today try eating dried apricots between your school classes. At the snack bar order a glass of juice (they might only have orange juice) and a plain cookie. When you get home, eat some crisp celery sticks. For your bedtime snack eat a piece of melon. Let's calculate the difference.

Just by making careful substitutions for your snacks you can save 883 calories in intake. To use up those extra 883 calories you would need to run fast

BEFORE		AFTER	
3, 1-OZ. CANDY BARS	150	4 HALVES DRIED APRICOTS	40
12 OZ. COKE	144	4 OZ. ORANGE JUICE	40
1 DOUGHNUT	176	CELERY STICKS	25
PEANUT BUTTER AND JELLY SANDWICH	263	1 PLAIN COOKIE	70
1 PC. CHOCOLATE CAKE	365	1 PC. MELON	40
TOTAL:	1098	TOTAL:	215

for about an hour and a half. Is it worth it? If you eat 883 fewer calories each day at the same energy expenditure, you would lose nearly two pounds of body fat in a week. So if you only need to lose twenty pounds of fat, you could do it in just ten weeks by substituting low-calorie snacks for your high-calorie snacks.

If you have more than twenty pounds to lose, you probably should plan and follow an exchange diet. If it is possible you should consult with a nutrition counselor or a dietician who can help you plan meals around your normal type of diet. If such counseling is not possible, read Chapter 9 on how to use exchange diets. With the help of your parent plan meals that will follow one of the exchange diets given in that chapter with addition of two milk exchanges. It is best if the entire family eats essentially the same meals as you do. (Members who do not need to lose weight can add extra exchanges of the given foods.) All members will benefit from a nutritious diet.

To learn which diet you should use, calculate the number of pounds that you wish to lose (probably your present weight minus your ideal weight). Each pound of fat is equivalent to about 3500 calories. Determine how fast you wish to lose the weight (no faster than two pounds per week). If you wish to lose two pounds per week, then you must eat 7000 fewer calories in the week than you are now eating, or use up extra calories with physical activity. To determine how many calories you now are eating, keep a food record for a week; calculate the calories for each day (from the number of exchanges); add the total calories for the week and divide by 7 to get the average number of calories per day. For example, if you consume 3000 calories per day and you want to lose two pounds per week, you need to consume 1000 calories less per day. This is probably too restrictive for a growing teen-ager; so a better way is to reduce your calories by, say, 500 and increase your activity to use up an extra 500 calories per day.

Let us now clarify a point of confusion for most people. Losing fat is not necessarily the same thing as losing weight. If you go on a very restrictive diet, without accompanying physical activity, you will lose weight, but part of that weight loss will be muscle protein loss—which you do not want. If you increase your physical activity while you are restricting your diet, the weight loss will be almost all fat. If you increase your physical activity, you will also be building more muscle tissue. Since muscle tissue weighs more than fat tissue, you can lose fat and gain muscle and weigh more than before you started the program. (But not for long.) Hence measuring weight loss is not the best way to determine the success of your program. A better criterion is to measure the inches lost. When you take a smaller dress size or you can pull your belt in another notch, then you know you are successful.

Another good criterion is how you look. As you replace flabby fat with firm muscles, you will look slimmer, and you will feel slimmer, even if your weight does not change. So don't worry about getting on the scales every morning. Instead notice how loose your clothes are becoming.

After you have succeeded in making substitutions for your snacks or in following a restrictive diet for a few weeks, you are ready for the third step in successful weight control. You probably are aware that you often eat when you are not really hungry. Maybe you eat because everyone else is eating. Or you eat because you are bored or lonely. The third step is to learn to substitute other activities for eating when you are not hungry.

Unless you can convince your friends to try some activity to substitute for their snack-bar visits, you probably will continue to eat at that time. This is okay if you will substitute a low-calorie food for a high-calorie one. Your biggest problem is probably when you are by yourself, either bored or lonely. What can you do as a diversion rather than eating? No, watching TV will not work. For too many people watching TV must be accompanied by food. Even if that isn't your habit, the commercials will quickly convince you that you need something to eat. If physical activity isn't possible or appropriate, try other diversionary activities—like phoning a friend, visiting a friend, washing the dishes, washing the car, taking a long bath, washing your hair—anything that takes your mind off eating until the urge passes. Make a list of things that you need to do, things that you like to do. Keep this list for emergencies when you are bored and lonely and want to eat. At that time select something from the list and do it instead of eating.

Now let us consider a couple of examples of two actual young people who learned to handle their overweight problems:

Debby was a somewhat pretty, 150-pound thirteen-year-old who had always been "chubby." She had a pleasing personality and was well liked by other children, so she had no motivation to try to lose weight. However, near the end of her eighth grade, she decided she wanted to be a cheerleader in high school, and she knew they didn't pick "fatties." Debby did not eat a great deal of food, but her physical activity was much less than normal. Debby did not like sports or PE and spent most of her free time watching TV or talking with her friends.

An analysis of Debby's typical daily energy intake and output revealed the following:

FOOD INTAKE

BREAKFAST	LUNCH	DINNER
1 C WHOLE MILK—1 MILK, FAT	1 HOT DOG—1 MEAT, 1 FAT	3 OZ. ROAST BEEF—3 MEAT, 3 FAT
2 SL. BREAD—2 BREAD	1 BUN—2 BREAD	2 TB. GRAVY—2 FAT, BREAD
2 TB. BUTTER—6 FAT	1 MILK SHAKE—1 MILK,	$\frac{1}{2}$ C PEAS—1 VEG.
2 TB. JELLY—2 SUGAR	2 FAT, 3 SUGAR	1 POTATO—2 BREAD
	2 COOKIES—1 SUGAR, 1 FAT	1 PC. CARAMEL CAKE—2 BREAD,
		3 FAT, $2\frac{1}{2}$ SUGAR
3 OZ. CANDY BAR—3 SUGAR,		
3 FAT, $1\frac{1}{2}$ BREAD	2 SL. BREAD—2 BREAD	
	4 TB. PEANUT BUTTER—4 FAT,	1 SL. BREAD—1 BREAD
	2 MEAT	2 TB. PEANUT BUTTER—1 MEAT,
		2 FAT
	4 TB. HONEY—4 SUGAR	2 TB. HONEY—2 SUGAR

TOTALS

EXCHANGES	CAL	PRO	CHO	FAT
2 MILK	160	16	24	—
7 MEAT	385	49	—	21
1 VEG.	25	2	5	—
0 FRUIT	0	0	0	0
$12\frac{1}{2}$ BREAD	875	25	187	—
29 FAT	1305	—	—	145
$17\frac{1}{2}$ SUGAR	840	—	210	—
	3590	92	426	166

ENERGY OUTPUT

WALKING, 100 MIN.	350 CAL.
CYCLING, 5 MIN.	25 CAL.
DAILY ACTIVITIES	800 CAL.
BASAL METABOLISM	2000 CAL.
	3175

As you will note, her energy intake was greater than her energy output. So the extra energy was stored as fat. Debby wanted to lose thirty pounds in four months, which is a reasonable two pounds per week. There would never be a better time in Debby's life for losing weight because from now on Debby's basal metabolism would continue to drop. Debby had a conference with her diet counselor and agreed to make the following changes:

1. To drink four glasses of milk each day to ensure an adequate supply of calcium, riboflavin, vitamin A, and vitamin D.
2. To cut down her sweets to one simple dessert each day.
3. To cut down her bread-and-peanut-butter snacks to one slice of bread with peanut butter and honey each day.
4. The rest of her snacks would consist of skim milk, fruit, or vegetables.
5. To increase her physical activity by 300 calories per day.

Debby made some changes in her life, but not very drastic changes. She continued eating three meals and three snacks a day; she continued eating the foods she liked, although in reduced quantities.

BREAKFAST	LUNCH	DINNER
1 C SKIM MILK—1 MILK	1 HOT DOG—1 MEAT, 1 FAT	3 OZ. ROAST BEEF—3 MEAT, 3 FAT
1 SL. WW. BREAD—1 BREAD	1 BUN—2 BREAD	1 POTATO—2 BREAD
$\frac{1}{2}$ TSP BUTTER—$\frac{1}{2}$ FAT	1 C SKIM MILK—1 MILK	1 TB. GRAVY—1 FAT, $\frac{1}{2}$ BREAD
1 EGG—1 MEAT, $\frac{1}{2}$ FAT	1 TOMATO—1 VEG.	1 C TOSSED SALAD—1 VEG.
$\frac{1}{2}$ C ORANGE JUICE—1 FRUIT		1 TB. SALAD DRESSING— 1 FAT
	1 SL. BREAD—1 BREAD	$\frac{1}{2}$ C PEAS—1 VEG.
4 DRIED APRICOTS—2 FRUIT	2 TB. PEANUT BUTTER—2 FAT, 1 MEAT	1 C SKIM MILK—1 MILK
	2 TB. HONEY—2 SUGAR	2 FIG BARS—2 SUGAR, $\frac{1}{2}$ BREAD
		1 C SKIM MILK—1 MILK
		1 BANANA—2 FRUIT

TOTALS

EXCHANGES	CAL	PRO	CHO	FAT
4 MILK	320	32	48	—
6 MEAT	330	42	—	18
9 FAT	405	—	—	45
7 BREAD	490	14	105	—
5 FRUIT	200	—	50	—
3 VEG.	75	6	15	—
4 SUGAR	192	—	48	—
	2012	94	266	63

ENERGY OUTPUT

WALKING, 3 MPH, 100 MIN.	350 CAL.
DAILY ACTIVITIES	800 CAL.
EXTRA ACTIVITIES	300 CAL.
BASAL METABOLISM	2000 CAL.
	3450 CAL.

ENERGY OUTPUT	3450 CAL.
FOOD INTAKE	2012 CAL.
DEFICIT	1438 CAL.

$$\frac{1438 \text{ CAL./DAY} \times 7 \text{ DAY}}{3500 \text{ CAL./LB.}} = 2.9 \text{ LB./WEEK}$$

Debby's major change was in the amount of physical activity she had. Rather than riding the bus, Debby and her best friend decided to ride their bikes to and from school for the rest of the school year. This required forty-four minutes, or 220 calories. In the evenings Debby and her sister set up a dancercise routine for twenty minutes each day. This used up about 80 calories.

Debby's new pattern of living was one that she could follow for a long time. She could still eat her meals with her family and friends, with only minor changes. Her cycling was to a required destination, and with a good friend, so that was easy to continue. Her dancercise with her sister was enough fun to make her want to keep it up.

Mike's problem was a little different. Mike had been teased whenever he tried to participate in sports for as long as he could remember: "Tubby can't run," "We don't want fatso on our team." As a result he spent most of his free time at home alone watching TV and munching on a candy bar. That is, until one day when he was fourteen, when his PE teacher said to him, "Mike, why don't you join the swim team? Your form is good, and with some training, you could be an excellent swimmer." (Mike's family had a backyard pool, so he had learned to swim fairly well when he was younger.) Mike hesitated at first, but he was reaching the age at which he desperately needed peer approval—perhaps he could get on the swim team.

The swim coach was very strict: "Follow the rules or get out!" The coach gave them a simple diet to follow, and said, "No junk food!" Each team member had to jog for thirty minutes each morning and attend swim practice for two hours each afternoon. Mike added an extra two-hour practice on Saturday morning.

For the first time in his life Mike was ravenously hungry. Between meals and after practice, before dinner, he ate apples, pears, bananas, oranges, cheese, nuts, whole-wheat crackers, skim milk—anything his mother had available for him. In a few months Mike not only won several blue ribbons at the swim meets, but he had also lost forty pounds.

At fourteen, Mike was just entering into his rapid-growth spurt. So in order to lose weight all he had to do was reduce his empty-calorie foods and greatly increase his physical activity. When Mike leaves school, if he will substitute some other activity for his swim team, he will be able to maintain a normal weight.

Debby and Mike were highly motivated; what about teen-agers who aren't? Let's review some principles of a teen-age weight-control program:

1. Because of the high energy requirement for growth, this is your easiest time to lose weight.
2. Your diet must include all the nutrients required for health and growth.
3. Increasing your physical activity is more important than decreasing your food intake.
4. Support of important persons—family, friends, teachers—is necessary to help you make the necessary changes.
5. Make small changes that you can live with for a long time.

Older teen-agers, who have passed their rapid-growth spurt, can profitably follow the weight-control program in this book. You can follow the basic weight-reduction diets exactly, with the addition of two milk exchanges to provide the necessary protein and calcium and vitamin D for growth.

CHAPTER 14

Weight Control During Pregnancy and Lactation

At last the long-awaited baby is on its way, but now you are afraid you are putting on too much weight. You've heard the old saying, "Twenty pounds for each baby," so you want to go on a diet. Let us state the first principle of weight control during pregnancy: *Pregnancy is not the time to lose weight.* If you are overweight, lose weight *before* you get pregnant, or wait until after the baby is born. But *never* try to lose weight during pregnancy. On the other hand pregnancy is not the time to eat everything to excess. Excess weight gain is also damaging to the fetus.

The components of average maternal weight gain are shown in the table on p. 142. If the mother's weight gain is less than the weight of the maternal components in pregnancy, the growth of the fetus calls on the reserves of the mother.

Very little weight should be gained during the first several weeks. Most of the weight should be gained during the last trimester of pregnancy. Figure 13 shows the amount of weight that should be gained each week of pregnancy. A gain of 1.5 to 3 pounds during the first trimester and a gain of about 0.8 pound per week during the remainder of pregnancy is considered ideal. A sudden gain in weight after the twentieth week may indicate water retention.

Tissue	Weight (lbs.)
Fetus	7.5
Uterus	2.0
Placenta	1.5
Amniotic Fluid	2.0
Blood Volume	3.0
Extracellular Fluid	2.0
Breast Tissue	1.0
Fat	9.0
TOTAL:	28.0

Components of Average Maternal Weight Gain

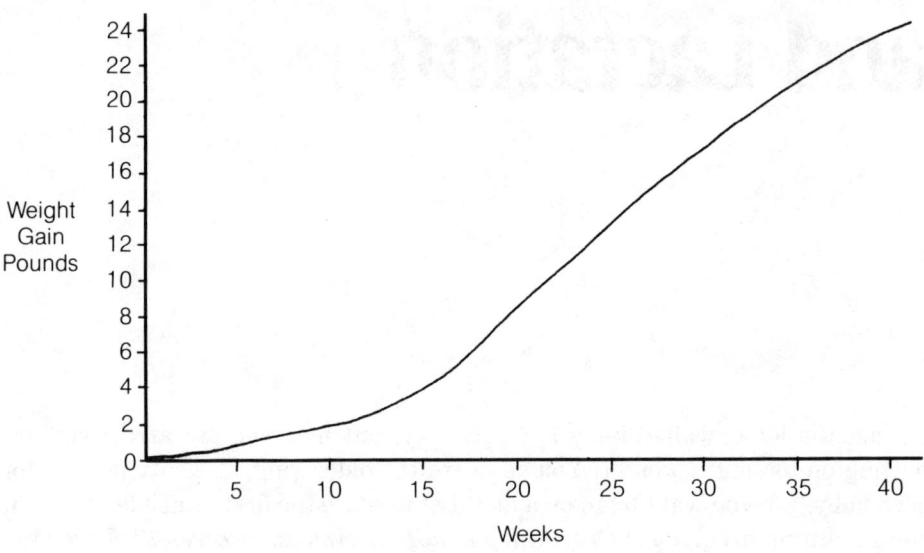

Fig. 13   Normal Curve of Weight Gain During Pregnancy

A recent government study followed the course of 53,518 pregnancies, and the subsequent course of the infants to eight years of age. A comprehensive analysis of the data from this study was made by Richard L. Naeye in 1979. This study showed that a mother's optimal weight gain in pregnancy—that gain that produced the fewest fetal and infant deaths—depends on her body build. The results of this study are summarized below:

Body Build	Optimum Weight Gain
Overweight Mothers	16 lbs.
Normal-weight Mothers	20 lbs.
Underweight Mothers	30 lbs.

For all three groups of mothers the fetal-mortality rates increased with weight gain less or more than these optimal values. Even large stores of body fat do not seem to ensure an optimal outcome of pregnancy when weight gains are very low, or when mothers lose weight. The results of this study indicate that the fetus may be more vulnerable to maternal dietary deficiencies and excesses than has often been assumed.

During pregnancy is the time to develop habits of good nutrition if these are not already established. Approximately 1800 to 2800 calories of carefully selected foods are necessary to meet the requirements for optimum growth of your baby. If you seem to be gaining too much weight, it is better to increase your physical activity than to restrict your calorie intake below 1800. Since during pregnancy your baby will have the greatest growth spurt of its entire life, this is the most important time for you to provide the optimum nutritional environment for your child. An inadequate diet may result in a stillborn, premature, or congenitally defective infant.

The first concern for an adequate diet is to obtain sufficient protein to provide the amino acids necessary for tissue building. It is recommended that you eat at least 75 grams of protein every day. Two thirds of the protein should come from meat, eggs, cheese, milk, poultry, and fish, since all the essential amino acids are provided by these foods. If your protein intake is inadequate, your baby will not be able to build the necessary tissues, and stunted growth and mental retardation may be the result. In addition, you may suffer from water retention, toxemia, anemia, and a lowered resistance to infection.

Calcium is one of the most important elements of your diet during pregnancy. If your diet is inadequate in calcium, you will sacrifice calcium from your bones to supply the needs of your child. This loss of calcium may lead to osteoporosis later in your life. Your infant requires approximately 30 grams of calcium before birth. It is recommended that your diet contain 1200 mg calcium daily.

Milk is one of the most important foods for the pregnant mother. Four cups of milk will supply the needed 1200 mg of calcium and will, in addition, supply the extra 30 grams of protein that you need. The milk will also supply the RDA for vitamins A and D if the milk is fortified. In addition, four cups of milk will supply the RDA for phosphorus and riboflavin.

A number of milk choices are available: whole milk, if you need to gain weight; skim or 2 percent milk, if you need to cut down calories. Other selections are buttermilk, yogurt, various cheeses, and (if made from milk) ice cream. If you find drinking milk distasteful, you may utilize the required amount in food dishes such as custards, puddings, and soups. Nonfat powdered milk can be added to dishes such as meat loaf, soups, mashed and scalloped potatoes, sandwich spreads, scrambled eggs, cooked cereals, homemade breads, cookies, pastries, cottage cheese, macaroni, or spaghetti. If you are lactose intolerant, you may be able to tolerate cheese, which contains only minute amounts of lactose. If you do not use sufficient milk or cheese, commercial supplements such as calcium lactate or calcium carbonate will supply the necessary calcium, but not the other nutrients in milk.

Many women have insufficient iron stores to meet the requirements of the growing child. The RDA is set at 18 mg daily, but this is very difficult to obtain from food only. The Food and Nutrition Board recommends a daily supplement of 30 to 60 mg ferrous iron daily during the second and third trimesters of pregnancy.

Iodine is of special importance during pregnancy because of its requirement for the hormone that helps control metabolism. An inadequate intake may result in goiter in both mother and child. In severe iodine deficiency your child may develop a type of mental retardation known as *cretinism.* Iodine supplements, usually as iodized salt, are recommended.

Folacin deficiency is probably the most common deficiency of pregnancy. During this time your folacin requirements are markedly increased because this is a period of rapid cell multiplication and DNA synthesis. The RDA of 800 μg daily usually cannot be met by diet alone. A daily folacin supplement of 400 to 800 μg is recommended.

Vitamin D is necessary for the absorption and utilization of calcium by both you and your child. If you are in the sunlight frequently each day, you can synthesize your own vitamin D. Otherwise you can obtain the RDA from four cups of fortified milk.

Linoleic acid, which is the one fatty acid essential for the unborn child, appears to be involved in the development of nerve tissue. Linoleic acid and vitamin E can both be obtained from oils, such as corn, soybean, or safflower.

Ascorbic acid (vitamin C) is another vitamin commonly deficient in the diet of pregnant women. Vitamin C is required for the formation of the connective tissue and vascular system of the baby. It is recommended that you eat at least two servings of citrus fruits, tomatoes, or green peppers to supply sufficient vitamin C.

Sometimes a mother is deficient in vitamin K, which is necessary for blood clotting. In these cases the infant is given vitamin K soon after birth to prevent hemorrhaging.

The exchange diet given below is suitable for both pregnancy and lactation. In the chart that follows, the nutrients in the exchange diet are compared with the RDAs for pregnancy and lactation.

In planning meals around the exchange diet for pregnancy and lactation it is important to use foods high in iron, such as liver, lean meats, deep green vegetables, and dried fruits. You should select two exchanges of citrus fruits or tomatoes and two or more exchanges of deep green, leafy vegetables or deep

Exchanges	CAL	PRO GRAMS	CHO GRAMS	FAT GRAMS	Calcium MG	Iron MG	Vit. A IU	Vit. D IU	Thi MG	Rib MG	Nia MG	Vit. C MG	Folacin MG
4 MILK	320	32	48	—	1368	0.4	416	400	.36	1.8	1.0	8	
6 MEAT	330	42	—	18	180	5.4	240	—	.54	0.6	7.8	2	
6 BREAD	420	12	90	—	95	4.5	2200	—	.40	0.3	4.0	15	
6 FRUIT	240	—	60	—	78	3.0	3678	—	.24	0.2	2.2	11	
4 VEG.	100	8	20	—	152	2.4	5913	—	.20	0.3	2.0	92	
9 FAT	405	—	—	45	*	*	*	*	*	*	*	*	*
TOTALS	1820	94	218	63	1873	15.7	12477	400	1.74	3.2	17	128	
PREGNANCY		74			1200	18	5000	400	1.4	1.5	15	80	0.8
LACTATION		64			1200	18	7000	400	1.5	1.7	18	70	0.5

Using the above exchange diet, we can plan meals such as the following:

BREAKFAST	LUNCH	DINNER
8 OZ. 2% MILK—1 MILK, 1 FAT 1 EGG—1 MEAT, ½ FAT 2 SL. WW. TOAST—2 BREAD 1 TSP. SOFT MARG.—1 UNSAT. FAT ½ GRAPEFRUIT—1 FRUIT	2 OZ. SKINLESS CHICKEN—2 MEAT 1 C TOSSED ROMAINE SALAD—1 VEG. 2 TSP. SALAD DRESSING—1 UNSAT. FAT 1 PC. CORNBREAD—1 BREAD, 1 FAT 12 GRAPES—1 FRUIT 8 OZ. SKIM MILK—1 MILK	2 OZ. LIVER W/ONIONS; COOKED IN OIL—2 MEAT, 1 UNSAT. FAT ½ C RICE—1 BREAD ½ C PEAS—1 BREAD ½ C SUMMER SQUASH—1 VEG. TOMATO AND CUCUMBER SLICES—1 VEG. 1 TSP. MAYONNAISE—1 UNSAT. FAT 4 OZ. GRAPE JUICE—2 FRUIT
SNACK	**SNACK**	**SNACK**
1 APPLE—1 FRUIT 1 SL. CHEESE—1 MEAT, 1 FAT	CARROT STICKS—1 VEG. 4 DRIED APRICOT HALVES—1 FRUIT 8 OZ. SKIM BUTTERMILK—1 MILK	8 OZ. 2% MILK—1 MILK, 1 FAT 1 PC. PLAIN CAKE—1 BREAD, 1 FAT

yellow vegetables. In addition, at least three of your fat exchanges should be from polyunsaturated oils, such as corn, soybean, sunflower, or safflower oils.

The above is a basic exchange diet. If you need more calories, you may eat any other foods that you desire. If you are overweight at the start of pregnancy, you should still eat the basic diet with the following modifications. Skim milk may be used instead of 2 percent or whole milk, and your fat exchanges may be reduced to three if you use only polyunsaturated oils. Pregnancy is a good time to avoid empty-calorie or extra-fuel foods.

And this is a good time to bring your attention to some very important "don'ts" of pregnancy: alcohol, tobacco, drinks containing caffeine, and diet drinks. For the sake of your unborn child you should totally abstain from alcohol and tobacco. You should drastically limit your consumption of drinks containing caffeine and saccharin. "Oh, no," you say, "that is too great a sacrifice." But look at it in perspective—your sacrifice is only for nine months; if you don't make the sacrifice, the damage to your child will last for his or her lifetime.

First and most important is the avoidance of alcoholic beverages. Continuing research is showing that alcohol consumption by pregnant women is the number one cause of mental retardation in children in the Western world. Alcohol crosses the placental barrier into the bloodstream of the infant and destroys the developing brain cells. One drink per day during half a pregnancy is sufficient to cause learning disabilities in a child. Five drinks per day is sufficient to cause the condition known as "fetal alcohol syndrome." In this condition the child is born with a smaller brain than normal, with defects in face and head structure, and with severe mental retardation. These defects are permanent and do not improve as the child grows older. A drunken mother usually has a hangover. That will pass away in a few hours. For the fetus the hangover may last a lifetime.

The question is frequently asked, "What is the safe level for alcohol consumption in the pregnant woman?" The most conservative answer given by medical authorities is that the thoughtful woman contemplating pregnancy would avoid all alcohol from the time of conception until the child is born.

The effects of maternal smoking on an unborn child are much less conclusive. They appear to be related to the decreased blood flow caused by smoking. Heavy smoking is associated with a greater incidence of miscarriages and low birth weight of infants. Some congenital deformities seem to be associated with heavy smoking. Also infants whose mothers smoke are more likely to be admitted to the hospital during the first year of life for pneumonia or bronchitis. The possibilities of damaging effects on the unborn child are great enough that a wise mother will cut down or cut out smoking.

It has been shown that nonsmokers who live with smokers and receive "second-hand" smoke have a greater risk of getting such lung diseases as bronchitis, pneumonia, emphysema, and lung cancer than do persons who are not exposed to smoke. Wise mothers and fathers will not allow their children, especially infants, to be exposed.

There is still much controversy regarding the effects of caffeine and saccharin on an unborn child. Probably the greatest problem is that a woman who is a heavy coffee, tea, or diet soda drinker is taking those drinks, which contain no nutrients, instead of milk or other food which do contain nutrients. A heavy coffee, tea, or diet soda drinker will probably have an inadequate intake of nutrients such as calcium, protein, riboflavin, vitamin A, and vitamin D.

Caffeine rapidly crosses the placental barrier into the bloodstream of the infant. Some of the biological effects of caffeine include a diuretic, a cardiac muscle stimulant, a smooth-muscle relaxant, and a stimulator of stomach-acid secretion. Whether or not these effects are detrimental to the child is not known with certainty. However, in animals caffeine hinders the development of bone and results in bone birth defects. There have been some reports of a link of coffee drinking with cancer; but these as yet are not substantiated.

The effects of saccharin are still controversial. However, the National Cancer Institute has recommended that in light of the present evidence saccharin should not be used at all by children or pregnant women. Since saccharin is currently the only nonnutritive sweetener permitted in diet drinks, such drinks are not recommended during pregnancy.

If you are gaining too much weight during pregnancy, the best thing to do is to increase your physical activity. A walking program is especially good at this time. Pregnancy is also a good time to practice your behavior modification techniques to improve your eating habits. You can drink skim milk rather than whole milk. You can reduce your fat exchanges to three, provided those three exchanges contain a good source of linoleic acid. But most important is to ensure the optimum growth and development environment for your child by consuming a nutritionally adequate diet.

After your baby is born, if you nurse the baby, you have your greatest opportunity to lose weight. Most infants require about 500 calories per day for the first three months and 600 to 700 calories per day from four to six months. That is equivalent to running fifty to seventy minutes every day! (You can't beat that.) Most nursing mothers can lose weight on the basic exchange diet for pregnancy (given on p. 145) since only 1100 to 1300 calories are available for the woman to use for herself. If you wish instead, you can follow the basic 1000-calorie diet (Chapter 9) for women, with the addition of two exchanges of milk to supply the extra calories, calcium, vitamin D, and protein needs for your baby.

After the birth of your baby is also a good time to increase your physical activity. Continue your walking program for the first few weeks. After your doctor gives approval, you can begin any of your aerobic exercises. This is also a good time to practice your toning exercises to help get your shape back to normal.

APPENDIX A.

Source Notes

Chapter 1. **What Makes People Fat?**

1. Most people keep a fairly stable weight after reaching middle age.

Sims, E.A.H., "Endocrine and Metabolic Effects of Experimental Obesity in Man," *Recent Progress in Hormone Research,* 29 (1973), 457.

"Morbid Obesity—Long Term Results in Therapeutic Fasting," *Nutrition Reviews,* 28 (1970), 216.

Margen, S., "Energy Balance with Increasing Weight," in *Obesity,* ed. N. L. Wilson (Philadelphia: F. A. Davis Co., 1969), p. 77.

2. Centers in the hypothalamus of the brain are thought to act like a furnace thermostat and hence are given the name *appestat.*

"The Feeding Center and Body Weight Reductions," *Nutrition Reviews,* 28 (1970), 216.

3. An appestat set too high is believed to be the cause of overweight in infants, adolescents, or in adults who suddenly gain much weight.

"Cellularity of Rat Adipose Tissue in Relation to Growth, Starvation and Obesity," *Nutrition Reviews,* 27 (1969), 1.

"Food and Obesity in the Rat," *Nutrition Reviews,* 37 (1979), 52.

4. There are three types of sensors that send signals to the appestat.

> Krause, M. V. and L. K. Mahan, *Food, Nutrition and Diet Therapy* (Philadelphia: W. B. Saunders Company, 1979), pp. 554–556.

5. Signals from fat-storage cells seem to be controlled by a set-point.

> "Human Obesity and Adipocyte Function," *Nutrition Reviews,* 36 (1978), 140.

6. Persons who are overfed in infancy or adolescence produce a greater than normal number of fat cells.

> "Cellularity of Rat Adipose Tissue," op. cit., p. 146.
>
> "Adipose Cell Size and Number in Experimental Human Obesity," *Nutrition Reviews,* 30, (1972), 60.
>
> "The Development of Adipose Tissue in Infancy," *Nutrition Reviews,* 37 (1979), 194.

7. The overproduction of insulin may be one cause of obesity. Research is now being conducted on ways to control the production of insulin.

> Albrink, M. J., "Dietary Fiber, Plasma, Insulin and Obesity," *American Journal of Clinical Nutrition,* 31 (1978), 5277.

8. Obesity in some persons may be caused by a deficiency of an enzyme that catalyzes many energy-using body reactions.

> "Some Obesity Tied to Key Enzyme Deficiency," *Chemical and Engineering News,* Nov. 10, 1980, p. 28.

9. In some persons a defect in brown-fat metabolism may be a cause of obesity.

> Danforth, E., "Dietary-Induced Thermogenesis: Control of Energy Expenditure," *Life Sciences,* 28 (1981), 1821–1827.

Chapter 2. **Walking the Tightrope**

1. A discussion of the U.S. RDAs.

> "1980 Revised Recommended Dietary Allowances," DIETETIC ASSOCIATION *American Journal,* 75 (1979), 623.

2. Source of food-composition information used in this book.

> U.S. Department of Agriculture, "The Nutritive Value of American Foods," Agriculture Handbook no. 456, Washington, D.C.: U.S. GPO, 1975.

3. Source of information on the water balance of a healthy person.

> Krause, op. cit., p. 187.

4. Temporary side effects have been reported from large doses of water-soluble vitamin pills.

> Krause, op. cit., p. 147.

5. Ascorbic acid appears to be one of the least toxic substances known.

> Pauling, L., "Ascorbic Acid and the Common Cold: Evaluation of its Efficacy and Toxicity," *Medical Tribune*, March 24, 1976.

6. Toxic effects of vitamins A and D have been reported.

> Krause, op. cit., p. 187.

7. Calcium deficiency is implicated in a fragile-bone disease known as osteoporosis.

> Heany, R. P., et al., "Calcium Balance and Calcium Requirements in Middle-Age Women," *American Journal of Clinical Nutrition*, 30 (1977), 1603.
>
> Jowsey, J., "Osteoporosis: Its Nature and Role of Diet," *Postgraduate Medicine*, 60 (1976), 78.

8. High-sodium diets may be a cause of essential hypertension.

> Cullen, R. W., et al., "Sodium, Hypertension, and the U.S. Dietary Goals," *Journal of Nutrition Education*, 10 (1978), 59.

9. Diets that contain two times the RDA of protein have been shown to cause a loss of blood calcium.

> Allen, U. A., et al., "Protein-Induced Hypercaliuria: A Long-Term Study," *American Journal of Clinical Nutrition*, 32 (1979), 741.

10. High-fiber diets are effective in promoting weight reduction.

> Van Itallie, T. B., "Fiber and Obesity," *American Journal of Clinical Nutrition*, 31 (1978), S-252.
>
> Heaton, K. W., et al., "How Fiber May Prevent Obesity," *American Journal of Clinical Nutrition*, 31 (1978), S-280.

11. Source for dietary goals.

> U.S. Senate Select Committee on Nutrition and Human Needs, *Dietary Goals for the United States*, 2nd ed., Washington, D.C.: U.S. GPO, 1977.

Chapter 3. **Meat Pies to Muscles**

1. Meal-fed rats become more obese than do nibbling rats.

> "Metabolic Changes in Meal-Fed Rats," *Nutrition Reviews*, 28 (1970), 23.

2. During moderate activity muscles "burn" fatty acids; during strenuous activity,

muscles "burn" glucose anaerobically.

"Exercise, Nutrition and Caloric Sources for Energy," *Nutrition Reviews,* 28 (1970), 182.

Alexander, R. M. and G. Goldspink, eds., *Mechanics and Energetics of Animal Locomotion* (London: Chapman & Hall 1977), p. 58.

Issekutz, B., Jr., "Energy Mobilization in Exercising Dogs," *Diabetes,* 28 Supplement 1 (1979), 39.

Chapter 4. **The Triple Bonus**

1. Source for Figure 11.

   Krause, op. cit., p. 26.

2. Source for Table 4.

   Margen, op. cit., p. 81.

3. Source for Table 4-2.

   Allsen, P. E., J. M. Harrison and B. Vance, *Fitness for Life,* (Dubuque, Iowa: William C. Brown Company, 1976), pp. 89–93.

4. Inactivity leads to muscle loss, fat gain, and more inactivity. Physical activity will reverse this vicious cycle.

   Leon, A. S., et al., "Effects of a Vigorous Walking Program on Body Composition, and Carbohydrate and Lipid Metabolism of Obese Young Men," *American Journal of Clinical Nutrition,* 32 (1979), 1776.

   Hanley, D. F., Jr., "Athletic Training and How Diet Affects It," *Nutrition Today,* 14 (1979), 5.

5. The physiological effects of inactivity result in many clinical diseases.

   Robbin, A. F., "The Exercise Prescription," *Obesity & Bariatric Medicine,* 2 (1973), 26.

   Stuart, R. B., "Exercise Prescription in Weight Management," *Obesity & Bariatric Medicine,* 4 (1975), 16.

   Morehouse, L. E., and A. T. Miller, *The Physiology of Exercise* (St. Louis: The C. V. Mosby Co., 1963), p. 70.

6. Another bonus is the "runner's high."

   Haier, R. S., et al., "Naloxone Alters Pain Perception After Jogging," *Psychiatry Research,* in press.

Chapter 5. **The Devil Made Me Do It**

1. Principles of behavior modification.

> Badura, A., *Principles of Behavior Modification* (New York: Holt, Rinehart and Winston, Inc., 1969).

Chapter 6. Fad Diets—Solutions or Illusions?

1. Fasting, without accompanying muscle activity, result in loss of both muscle and fat tissue; resumption of eating replaces only fat tissue.

> Young, D. R., *Physical Performance, Fitness and Diet* (Springfield, Ill.: Charles C. Thomas, 1977).
>
> "Morbid Obesity," op. cit., p. 216.

2. Recommendations for use of liquid-protein diets.

> "Caveat Dieter," *Chemistry,* 51(6) (1978), 25.
>
> "Liquid Protein Diets," *U.S. News & World Report,* October 20, 1980, p. 84.

3. Critique on low-carbohydrate diets.

> Council on Foods and Nutrition, "A Critique of Low-Carbohydrate Ketogenic Weight Reduction Regimens," *Journal of the American Medical Association,* 224 (10) (1973).

4. Ketone bodies are known to cause brain damage to a developing fetus.

> "Maternal Weight Gain and the Outcome of Pregnancy," *Nutrition Reviews,* 37 (1979), 318.

5. Source for Table 7 and Figure 12.

> Yang, M. U. and T. B. Van Itallie, "Composition of Weight Loss During Short-Term Weight Reduction," *Journal of Clinical Investigation,* 58 (1976), 722.

6. A balanced diet results in a greater long-term fat loss than does starvation or a ketogenic diet.

> Lewis, S. B., et al., "Effect of Diet Composition on Metabolic Adaptations to Hypocaloric Nutrition," *American Journal of Clinical Nutrition,* 30 (1977), 160.

7. The weight loss on a 500-calorie diet with HCG is no different than on a 500-calorie diet without HCG.

> Chlouverakis, C. S., "Facts and Fancies in Weight Control, (III)—The Fat That Does Not Melt Away," *Obesity & Bariatric Medicine,* 4 (1975), 164.

8. Side effects of HCG.

> F. Stare, "Dr. Fred Stare Rates the Ten Top Diets," *Harper's Bazaar,* July 1977, p. 40.

9. Recommendations for bypass surgery.

"Use of Intestinal Bypass to Treat Morbid Obesity," *Nutrition Reviews,* 35 (1977), 172.

Chapter 9. **Getting There**

1. Source of original exchange list.

"Exchange Lists for Meal Planning," American Diabetes Association, Inc., The American Dietetic Association, 1978.

2. Source for Table 9.

Davis, D. R., "Wheat and Nutrition," *Nutrition Today,* Sept./Oct. 1981, pp. 22–25.

3. Source for nutrient composition of exchange groups.

Wyse, B. A., "Nutrient Analysis of Exchanges Lists for Meal Planning," *Journal of the American Dietetic Association,* 75 (1978), 238.

4. Saccharin may be hazardous to your health.

Hoover, R., "Saccharin," *New England Journal of Medicine,* March 6, 1980, p. 573.

5. The effects of caffeine on humans.

"Third International Caffeine Workshop," *Nutrition Reviews,* 39 (1981), 183.

6. There is some evidence that six meals are more conducive to weight loss than three meals.

"Metabolic Changes in Meal-Fed Rats," op. cit., p. 23.

"Effects of Meal Frequency During Weight Reduction," *Nutrition Reviews,* 30 (1972), 158.

Chapter 10. **Getting There Faster**

1. A medical checkup is recommended before beginning an exercise program.

Cooper, K. H., *The New Aerobics,* (New York: M. Evans & Co., 1970), p. 22.

2. The maximum heart rate was determined by research.

Wilmore, J. H., and L. Haskell, "Use of the Heart Rate-Energy Expenditure Relationship in the Individualized Prescription of Exercise," *American Journal of Clinical Nutrition,* 24 (1971), 1186.

Chapter 13. **Weight Control in Adolescence**

Source for tables.
> Krause, op. cit., Ch. 15.

Chapter 14. **Weight Control During Pregnancy and Lactation**

1. Source for Figure 14.
> Krause, op. cit., p. 279.

2. Source for Figure 15.
> Ibid., p. 281.

3. An extensive study was made of maternal weight gain.
> Naeye, R. L., "Weight Gain and the Outcome of Pregnancy," *American Journal of Obstetrics and Gynecology,* 135 (1979), 3.

4. Unsaturated fatty acids are necessary for myelin formation in brain tissue.
> Baker, R.W.R., et al., "Fatty Acid Composition of Brain Lecithins in Multiple Sclerosis," *Lancet,* 1 (1963), 26.

5. Fetal alcohol syndrome.
> Iber, F. I., "Fetal Alcohol Syndrome," *Nutrition Today,* 15 (1980), 4.
> Enloe, F. F., "How Alcohol Affects the Developing Fetus," *Nutrition Today,* 15 (1980), 11.

APPENDIX B.
Charts and Tables

TABLE 12 RECOMMENDED DIETARY ALLOWANCES, REVISED 1980*

DESIGNED FOR THE MAINTENANCE OF GOOD NUTRITION OF PRACTICALLY ALL HEALTHY PEOPLE IN THE U.S.A.
FOOD AND NUTRITION BOARD, NATIONAL ACADEMY OF SCIENCES-NATIONAL RESEARCH COUNCIL

AGE AND SEX GROUP	WEIGHT KG	WEIGHT LB	HEIGHT CM	HEIGHT IN	PROTEIN GM	FAT-SOLUBLE VITAMINS — VITAMIN A (μG R.E.†)	VITAMIN D (μG‡)	VITAMIN E (MG αT.E.#)	WATER-SOLUBLE VITAMINS — VITAMIN C (MG)	THIAMIN (MG)	RIBOFLAVIN (MG)	NIACIN (MG N.E.¶)	VITAMIN B6 (MG)	FOLACIN (μG)	VITAMIN B12 (μG)	MINERALS — CALCIUM (MG)	PHOSPHORUS	MAGNESIUM	IRON	ZINC	IODINE (μG)
INFANTS																					
0.0–0.5 YR.	6	13	60	24	KG×2.2	420	10	3	35	0.3	0.4	6	0.3	30	0.5	360	240	50	10	3	40
0.5–1.0 YR.	9	20	71	28	KG×2.0	400	10	4	35	0.5	0.6	8	0.6	45	1.5	540	360	70	15	5	50
CHILDREN																					
1–3 YR.	13	29	90	35	23	400	10	5	45	0.7	0.8	9	0.9	100	2.0	800	800	150	15	10	70
4–6 YR.	20	44	112	44	30	500	10	6	45	0.9	1.0	11	1.3	200	2.5	800	800	200	10	10	90
7–10 YR.	28	62	132	52	34	700	10	7	45	1.2	1.4	16	1.6	300	3.0	800	800	250	10	10	120
MALES																					
11–14 YR.	45	99	157	62	45	1,000	10	8	50	1.4	1.6	18	1.8	400	3.0	1,200	1,200	350	18	15	150
15–18 YR.	66	145	176	69	56	1,000	10	10	60	1.4	1.7	18	2.0	400	3.0	1,200	1,200	400	18	15	150
19–22 YR.	70	154	177	70	56	1,000	7.5	10	60	1.5	1.7	19	2.2	400	3.0	800	800	350	10	15	150
23–50 YR.	70	154	178	70	56	1,000	5	10	60	1.4	1.6	18	2.2	400	3.0	800	800	350	10	15	150
51+ YR.	70	154	178	70	56	1,000	5	10	60	1.2	1.4	16	2.2	400	3.0	800	800	350	10	15	150
FEMALES																					
11–14 YR.	46	101	157	62	46	800	10	8	50	1.1	1.3	15	1.8	400	3.0	1,200	1,200	300	18	15	150
15–18 YR.	55	120	163	64	46	800	10	8	60	1.1	1.3	14	2.0	400	3.0	1,200	1,200	300	18	15	150
19–22 YR.	55	120	163	64	44	800	7.5	8	60	1.1	1.3	14	2.0	400	3.0	800	800	300	18	15	150
23–50 YR.	55	120	163	64	44	800	5	8	60	1.0	1.2	13	2.0	400	3.0	800	800	300	18	15	150
51+ YR.	55	120	163	64	44	800	5	8	60	1.0	1.2	13	2.0	400	3.0	800	800	300	10	15	150
PREGNANCY					+30	+200	+5	+2	+20	+0.4	+0.3	+2	+0.6	+400	+1.0	+400	+400	+150	††	+5	+25
LACTATION					+20	+400	+5	+3	+40	+0.5	+0.3	+5	+0.5	+100	+1.0	+400	+400	+150	††	+10	+50

† 1 μg R.E. equals 5 IU vitamin A.

‡ 1 μg equals 40 IU vitamin D.

¶ 1 N.E. (niacin equivalent) equals 1 mg niacin or 60 mg dietary tryptophan (from protein).

†† The increased requirement during pregnancy cannot be met by the diets of most Americans; therefore the use of 30 to 60 mg supplemental iron is recommended.

ESTIMATED SAFE AND ADEQUATE DAILY DIETARY INTAKES OF ADDITIONAL SELECTED VITAMINS AND MINERALS*

AGE GROUP	VITAMINS			TRACE ELEMENTS						ELECTROLYTES		
	VITAMIN K	BIOTIN	PANTOTHENIC ACID	COPPER	MANGANESE	FLUORIDE	CHROMIUM	SELENIUM	MOLYBDENUM	SODIUM	POTASSIUM	CHLORIDE
	µG			MG								
INFANTS												
0.0–0.5 YR.	12	35	2	0.5–0.7	0.5–0.7	0.1–0.5	0.01–0.04	0.01–0.04	0.03–0.06	115– 350	350– 925	275– 700
0.5–1.0 YR.	10– 20	50	3	0.7–1.0	0.7–1.0	0.2–1.0	0.02–0.06	0.02–0.06	0.04–0.08	250– 750	425–1,275	400–1,200
CHILDREN AND ADOLESCENTS												
1–3 YR.	15– 30	65	3	1.0–1.5	1.0–1.5	0.5–1.5	0.02–0.08	0.02–0.08	0.05–0.1	325– 975	550–1,650	500–1,500
4–6 YR.	20– 40	85	3–4	1.5–2.0	1.5–2.0	1.0–2.5	0.03–0.12	0.03–0.12	0.06–0.15	450–1,350	775–2,325	700–2,100
7–10 YR.	30– 60	120	4–5	2.0–2.5	2.0–3.0	1.5–2.5	0.05–0.2	0.05–0.2	0.10–0.30	600–1,800	1,000–3,000	925–2,775
11+ YR.	50–100	100–200	4–7	2.0–3.0	2.5–5.0	1.5–2.5	0.05–0.2	0.05–0.2	0.15–0.5	900–2,700	1,525–4,575	1,400–4,200
ADULTS	70–140	100–200	4–7	2.0–3.0	2.5–5.0	1.5–4.0	0.05–0.2	0.05–0.2	0.15–0.5	1,100–3,300	1,875–5,625	1,700–5,400

*Since the toxic levels for many trace elements may be only several times usual intakes, the upper levels for the trace elements given in this table should not be habitually exceeded.

SOURCE: Reproduced from: Recommended Dietary Allowances, Ninth Revised Edition (1980, in press), with the permission of the National Academy of Sciences, Washington, D.C. J Am Diet Assoc Vol 75, Dec 1979 p 623.

FOOD EXCHANGES

MILK EXCHANGE
(ONE MILK EXCHANGE IS DEFINED AS 8 OZ. SKIM MILK OR ITS EQUIVALENT.)

ONE EXCHANGE OF MILK CONTAINS 12 GRAMS CARBOHYDRATE, 8 GRAMS PROTEIN, AND 80 CALORIES.

8	OZ. SKIM OR NONFAT MILK
1/3	CUP POWDERED, INSTANT, NONFAT, DRY MILK
¼	CUP POWDERED, REGULAR, NONFAT, DRY MILK
½	CUP CANNED, EVAPORATED SKIM MILK
1	CUP BUTTERMILK FROM SKIM MILK
1	CUP YOGURT FROM SKIM MILK (0 GRAMS FAT), PLAIN, UNFLAVORED (HOME RECIPE)
1	CUP CHOCOLATE MILK FROM SKIM MILK (1 MILK + 1 FAT + 1 BREAD)
8	OZ. 1% FAT-FORTIFIED MILK (1 MILK + ½ FAT)
8	OZ. 2% FAT-FORTIFIED (LOW-FAT) MILK (1 MILK + 1 FAT)
1	CUP LOW-FAT YOGURT (5 GRAMS FAT), PLAIN, UNFLAVORED (1 MILK + 1 FAT)
1	CUP LOW-FAT YOGURT, FLAVORED (1 MILK + 1 FAT + 1 SUGAR)
8	OZ. WHOLE MILK (1 MILK + 2 FAT)
½	CUP CANNED, EVAPORATED WHOLE MILK (1 MILK + 2 FAT)
1	CUP BUTTERMILK FROM WHOLE MILK (1 MILK + 2 FAT)
½	CUP CANNED, CONDENSED, SWEETENED MILK (1 MILK + 2 FAT + 6 SUGAR)
1	CUP CHOCOLATE MILK FROM WHOLE MILK (1 MILK + 3 FAT + 1 BREAD)
1	CUP ICE CREAM (1 MILK + 3 FAT + 1 SUGAR)
1	CUP SOFT SERVE ICE CREAM (1 MILK + 3½ FAT + 2 SUGAR)
1	CUP ICE MILK (1 MILK + 1 FAT + 1½ SUGAR)
1	CUP SOFT SERVE ICE MILK (1 MILK + 1½ FAT + 2½ SUGAR)
1	CUP MALTED MILK (1 MILK + 2 FAT)
1	CUP MILK SHAKE (1 MILK + 3 FAT)
1	CUP SOYBEAN MILK (1 MILK + 1 FAT)

MEAT EXCHANGE
(1 MEAT EXCHANGE IS DEFINED AS 1 OZ. LEAN MEAT [3 GRAMS FAT OR LESS] OR ITS EQUIVALENT.)
(THE MEAT IN THIS EXCHANGE LIST MUST HAVE ALL SEPARABLE FAT REMOVED.)
(THE MEAT IS COOKED MEAT; RAW MEAT LOSES APPROXIMATELY ¼ WEIGHT IN COOKING.)

ONE MEAT EXCHANGE CONTAINS 7 GRAMS PROTEIN, 3 GRAMS FAT, AND 55 CALORIES.

BEEF, 1 OZ.

FLANK STEAK	TIP ROAST
BOTTOM ROUND STEAK	ARM POT ROAST
TOP ROUND STEAK	HEEL OF ROUND POT ROAST
SIRLOIN STEAK	STANDING RUMP POT ROAST
TENDERLOIN STEAK	DRIED BEEF
T-BONE STEAK, TRIMMED	BEEF HEART
PORTERHOUSE STEAK, TRIMMED	BEEF LIVER

VEAL, 1 OZ.

ARM STEAK	LOIN CHOPS
BLADE STEAK	RIB CHOPS
SIRLOIN STEAK	RUMP ROAST
CUTLETS, ROUND	SIRLOIN ROAST
VEAL HEART	VEAL LIVER

PORK, 1 OZ.

SIRLOIN	LOIN, CENTER CUT
PORK HEART	LEG STEAK (FRESH HAM)
PORK LIVER	HAM, RUMP PORTION

LAMB, 1 OZ.

LOIN CHOP	LAMB HEART

LEG ROAST   LAMB LIVER

POULTRY, 1 OZ.
(MEAT WITHOUT SKIN)

CHICKEN   CORNISH HEN
TURKEY   PHEASANT
POULTRY LIVERS

FISH, 1 OZ.

ANY FRESH OR FROZEN FISH, OR SHELLFISH
¼ CUP CANNED SALMON, TUNA, MACKEREL, CRAB, LOBSTER
   (DRAINED OR CANNED IN WATER)

CHEESE, 1 OZ.

1 OZ. (1 SL.) "SLIM" AMERICAN PROCESSED CHEESE
   (IF 3 GRAMS FAT OR LESS PER OUNCE)
¼ CUP DRY AND LOW-FAT COTTAGE CHEESE

EGGS

2 EGG WHITES (0 GRAMS FAT)

LEGUMES

½ CUP COOKED DRIED BEANS, PEAS, LENTILS (1 MEAT + 1 BREAD)

MISCELLANEOUS

9 CUBES, 1½ OZ., OR 1 CUP BOUILLON CUBES
½ CAN (5 OZ.) CONSOMME SOUP

MEDIUM-FAT MEAT. ONE EXCHANGE CONTAINS 1 MEAT + ½ FAT; OR 7 GRAMS PROTEIN, 5½ GRAMS FAT, AND 78 CALORIES.

BEEF, 1 OZ.

TOP LOIN STEAK	RIB ROAST
RIB STEAK	CHUCK ROAST
CLUB STEAK	BLADE POT ROAST
GROUND ROUND	STEW MEAT, ROUND
CORNED BEEF	FRIED LIVER

PORK, 1 OZ.

BLADE STEAK	TENDERLOIN ROAST
BLADE (BOSTON) SHOULDER ROAST	CANADIAN BACON
ARM PICNIC SHOULDER ROAST	BOILED HAM
HAM, SHANK ROAST	FRIED LIVER

LAMB, 1 OZ.

ARM-BLADE CHOP	FRIED LIVER

CHEESE, 1 OZ.

MOZZARELLA	NEUFCHATEL
RICOTTA	3 TB GRATED PARMESAN
FARMER'S	¼ C CREAMED COTTAGE CHEESE

EGGS

1 WHOLE LARGE EGG

LEGUMES

1/3 CUP COOKED SOYBEANS (1 MEAT + ½ BREAD + ½ FAT)
3½ OZ. TOFU (1 MEAT + ½ FAT)

HIGH-FAT MEAT. ONE EXCHANGE CONTAINS 1 MEAT + 1 FAT; OR 7 GRAMS PROTEIN, 8 GRAMS FAT, AND 100 CALORIES.

BEEF, 1 OZ.

BRISKET
CORNED BEEF BRISKET
HAMBURGER, COMMERCIAL

GROUND BEEF
GROUND CHUCK

VEAL, 1 OZ.

STEW MEAT

BREAST

PORK, 1 OZ.

SMOKED ARM PICNIC ROAST
LOIN (BACK RIBS)
SPARE RIBS
GROUND PORK

COUNTRY-STYLE HAM
DEVILED HAM
SALAMI
2 OZ. SAUSAGE (1 MEAT + 2 FAT)
2 OZ. FRANKFURTERS (1 MEAT + 2 FAT)

COLD CUTS, 1 SLICE 4½" × ⅛"

LAMB, 1 OZ.

RIB CHOP

RIBLETS (BREAST)

POULTRY, 1 OZ.

ANY POULTRY WITH SKIN
CAPON
DUCK (DOMESTIC)

GOOSE
2 OZ. CHICKEN FRANKFURTERS
 (1 MEAT + 2 FAT)

CHEESE, 1 OZ.

CHEDDAR, ROQUEFORT, BLUE, SWISS, AMERICAN PROCESS CHEESE
 (1 SL., A 1" CUBE, OR ¼ CUP GRATED)

MISCELLANEOUS

COLD CUTS, MIXED MEATS, 1 SL., 4½" × ⅛"
2 TB. PEANUT BUTTER (1 MEAT + 2 FAT)
1 10½-OZ. CAN CREAM OF CHICKEN SOUP, CONDENSED (1 MEAT + 2 FAT)
1 C SHELLED NUTS: ALMONDS (3½ MEAT, 14 FAT, 1½ BREAD)
              PEANUTS (5 MEAT, 14 FAT, 2 BREAD)
              WALNUTS (2 MEAT, 13 FAT, 1 BREAD)

BREAD-CEREAL-STARCHY VEGETABLE EXCHANGE

ONE EXCHANGE CONTAINS 15 GRAMS CARBOHYDRATE, 2 GRAMS PROTEIN, AND 70 CALORIES.

BREAD: 28 GRAMS. 1 SL. COMMERCIAL WHITE, FRENCH, ITALIAN, WHOLE WHEAT,
                    RYE, PUMPERNICKEL, OR RAISIN
           ½ SL. HOMEMADE WHITE OR WHOLE WHEAT

½	SM. BAGEL
½	ENGLISH MUFFIN, SM.
1	PLAIN BREAD ROLL
½	HAMBURGER OR FRANKFURTER BUN
½	8" TORTILLA
1	TACO SHELL
½	CUP DRIED BREAD CRUMBS
1/3	CUP BREAD STUFFING MIX (1 BREAD + ½ FAT)
1	BISCUIT, 2" DIA. (1 BREAD + 1 FAT)
1	P. CORN BREAD, 2"×2"×1" (1 BREAD + 1 FAT)
1	SMALL MUFFIN, PLAIN (1 BREAD + 1 FAT)
½	DANISH PASTRY (1 BREAD + 1½ FAT)
1	PANCAKE, 5"×½" (1 BREAD + ½ FAT)
1	WAFFLE, 5"×½" (1 BREAD + ½ FAT)

CRACKERS, COOKIES
   3   ARROWROOT

2	GRAHAM, 2½" SQUARE
½	MATZOTH, 4"×6"
20	OYSTER
25	PRETZELS
3	RYE WAFERS, 2"×3½"
6	SALTINES
4	SODA, 2½" SQUARE
	CROUTONS
1	OATMEAL COOKIE (1 BREAD + ½ FAT + ½ SUGAR)
1	VANILLA WAFER (1 BREAD + ½ FAT + ½ SUGAR)
1	PLAIN SUGAR COOKIE (1 BREAD + ½ FAT + ½ SUGAR)

CAKES, PIES, DOUGHNUTS

1¼"	ARC ANGEL FOOD CAKE
2"	ARC SPONGE CAKE (1 BREAD + ½ FAT)
2½"	CUPCAKE, PLAIN, NO ICING (1 BREAD + 1 FAT)
1¾"	DIA. CREAM PUFF (1 BREAD + 2 FAT)
1	CAKE DOUGHNUT (1 BREAD + 1½ FAT + ½ SUGAR)
1	YEAST DOUGHNUT (1 BREAD + 2 FAT + ½ SUGAR)
1/12	APPLE PIE (1 BREAD + 2 FAT + 1 SUGAR)
1/12	BANANA CREAM PIE (1 BREAD + 1½ FAT + 1 SUGAR)
1/12	MINCE PIE (1 BREAD + 2 FAT + 1½ SUGAR)
1/12	PUMPKIN PIE (1 BREAD + 2 FAT + 1 SUGAR)

CEREAL-PASTA

½	CUP BRAN FLAKES
¾	CUP OTHER READY-TO-EAT CEREALS (UNSWEETENED)
¾	CUP READY-TO-EAT CEREALS, SWEETENED (1 BREAD + 1 SUGAR)
1	CUP PUFFED CEREAL (UNFROSTED)
½	CUP COOKED CEREAL, GRITS
½	CUP SPAGHETTI, NOODLES, MACARONI, OR RICE (COOKED)
	(1 LB. RAW RICE 3 C COOKED RICE 6 EXCHANGES)
	(1 LB. RAW SPAGHETTI 10½ C COOKED SPAGHETTI 20.8 EXCHANGES)
	(1 LB. RAW MACARONI 8.8 C COOKED MACARONI 17.6 EXCHANGES)
	(1 LB. RAW NOODLES 8.8 C COOKED NOODLES 17.8 EXCHANGES)
3	CUPS POPPED POPCORN, NO FAT ADDED

FLOURS

2	TB. CORNMEAL, DRY; OR ¼ CUP
2½	TB. WHEAT FLOUR; OR ABOUT ¼ CUP
2	TB. CORNSTARCH
3	TB. CAROB FLOUR
5	TB. COCOA, DRY (1 BREAD + 1 FAT)
1/3	CUP GRAHAM CRACKER CRUMBS

STARCHY VEGETABLES

1/3	CUP CORN OR 1 SM. COB OF CORN
½	CUP LIMA BEANS
2/3	CUP PARSNIPS
½	CUP GREEN PEAS (CANNED, FRESH, OR FROZEN)
1	SM. WHITE POTATO OR ½ CUP MASHED POTATOES
½	CUP WINTER, ACORN, OR BUTTERNUT SQUASH
¾	CUP PUMPKIN
¼	CUP YAM OR SWEET POTATO
½	OF 10½ OZ. CAN CREAM OF CELERY SOUP (1 BREAD + 2 FAT)
½	OF 10½ OZ. CAN CREAM OF MUSHROOM SOUP (1 BREAD + 1½ FAT)
½	OF 10½ OZ. CAN CREAM OF TOMATO SOUP (1 BREAD + ½ FAT)

FRUIT EXCHANGES

ONE EXCHANGE OF FRUIT CONTAINS 10 GRAMS CARBOHYDRATE AND 40 CALORIES

1	SM. APPLE, 2" DIAMETER.................................92 GRAMS OR 3 OZ.
1/3	CUP UNSWEETENED APPLE
2	MED. APRICOTS, FRESH.................................76 GRAMS OR 2¾ OZ.

4	HALVES, DRIED APRICOTS		
½	SM. BANANA, 7½"×1½"	70	GRAMS OR 2½ OZ.
1/5	CUP MASHED BANANAS		
½	CUP BLACKBERRIES		
½	CUP BLUEBERRIES		
10	LARGE CHERRIES	75	GRAMS OR 2¾ OZ.
¼	SM. CANTALOUPE, 5" DIAMETER		
2	DATES		
1	FIG, FRESH OR DRIED		
½	GRAPEFRUIT, 3½" DIAMETER		
½	CUP GRAPEFRUIT JUICE		
10	GRAPES, THOMPSON, SEEDLESS	50	GRAMS OR 1¾ OZ.
20	GRAPES, CONCORD	80	GRAMS OR 2¾ OZ.
¼	CUP GRAPE JUICE		
1/10	HONEYDEW MELON, 6½" DIAMETER		
¼	SM. MANGO		
½	NECTARINE, 2½" DIAMETER	75	GRAMS OR 2¾ OZ.
1	SM. ORANGE, 2½" DIAMETER	131	GRAMS OR 4¾ OZ.
½	CUP ORANGE JUICE		
¾	CUP PAPAYA		
2	PASSION FRUIT		
1	PEACH, 2½" DIAMETER	115	GRAMS OR 4⅛ OZ.
1	SM. PEAR, 2"×1½"	72	GRAMS OR 2½ OZ
1	MED. PERSIMMON, 2½" DIAMETER		
½	CUP PINEAPPLE		
1/3	CUP PINEAPPLE JUICE		
2	ITALIAN PLUMS	60	GRAMS OR 2⅛ OZ.
½	POMEGRANATE, 3½"×2½"	138	GRAMS OR 4⅞ OZ.
2	PRUNES		
¼	CUP PRUNE JUICE		
½	CUP RASPBERRIES		
2	TB. RAISINS	18	GRAMS OR .6 OZ.
¾	CUP STRAWBERRIES		
1	MED. TANGERINE, 2½" DIAMETER	116	GRAMS OR 4⅛ OZ.
1	CUP DICED WATERMELON		
1	PC. WATERMELON, 10" DIA., ½" THICK	463	GRAMS OR 16½ OZ.
1	TB. DARK OR BLACKSTRAP MOLASSES		
½	CUP LEMON JUICE		

VEGETABLE EXCHANGES
ONE EXCHANGE CONTAINS 5 GRAMS CARBOHYDRATE, 2 GRAMS PROTEIN, AND 25 CALORIES.

ONE VEGETABLE EXCHANGE IS 1 CUP RAW VEGETABLES OR ½ CUP COOKED VEGETABLES.

ARTICHOKES	CAULIFLOWER	MUSHROOMS	SUMMER SQUASH
ASPARAGUS	CELERY	MUSTARD GREENS	TOMATOES
BEAN SPROUTS	CHARD	OKRA	TOMATO JUICE
BEETS	COLLARDS	ONIONS	TURNIPS
BEET GREENS	CUCUMBER	RHUBARB	TURNIP GREENS
BROCCOLI	DANDELION GREENS	RUTABAGA	VEGETABLE JUICE
BRUSSELS SPROUTS	EGGPLANT	SAUERKRAUT	WATER CHESTNUTS
CABBAGE	GREEN PEPPER	SPINACH	ZUCCHINI
CARROTS	KALE	STRING BEANS	

RAW, WHOLE VEGETABLES: (ONE EXCHANGE EACH)

1	CARROT, 6¼"×1⅛"	67	GRAMS OR 2 OZ.
3	STICKS CELERY, 8"×1½"	120	GRAMS OR 4¼ OZ.
1	CUCUMBER, 8¼"×2"	175	GRAMS OR 6¼ OZ.
4	MED. GREEN ONIONS	60	GRAMS OR 2 OZ.
1	GREEN PEPPER, 2½"×2¼"	138	GRAMS OR 4⅞ OZ.

30   RADISHES, ¾″ DIA.................................. 150 GRAMS OR 5 1/3 OZ.
1   TOMATO, 2½″ DIA. .... 135 GRAMS OR 4¾ OZ.

1 CUP BAMBOO SHOOTS, CANNED   1 TB. DEHYD. ONION FLAKES
4 MED. DILL PICKLES   ½ SWEET PICKLE, GHERKIN

¼ OF A 10½ OZ. CAN CONDENSED ONION SOUP (1 VEG. + ½ FAT)
¼ OF A 10½ OZ. CAN CONDENSED TOMATO SOUP (1 VEG. + ½ BREAD + ½ FAT)

THE FOLLOWING RAW VEGETABLES MAY BE USED AS DESIRED:
CHICORY   ENDIVE   LETTUCE   RADISHES
CHINESE CABBAGE   ESCAROLE   PARSLEY   WATERCRESS

FAT EXCHANGES
ONE EXCHANGE OF FAT CONTAINS 5 GRAMS OF FAT AND 45 CALORIES.

COOKING FATS:
  POLYUNSATURATED:
    1 TSP. CORN OIL   1 TSP. SOYBEAN OIL
    1 TSP. COTTONSEED OIL   1 TSP. SUNFLOWER OIL
    1 TSP. SAFFLOWER OIL   1 TSP. SOFT OR LIQUID MARGARINE*
  MONOUNSATURATED:
    1 TSP. OLIVE OIL   1 TSP. PEANUT OIL
  SATURATED
    1 TSP. BUTTER   1 TSP. LARD
    1 TSP. BACON FAT   1 TSP. HARD MARGARINES
  DAIRY PRODUCTS: (SATURATED)
    2 TB. LIGHT CREAM   2 TB. SOUR CREAM, 4 TB. IMITATION SOUR CREAM
    1 TB. HEAVY CREAM   1 TB. CREAM CHEESE
  FRUITS: (MONOUNSATURATED)
    ⅛ AVOCADO, 4″ DIA.   5 SMALL OLIVES
  NUTS: (MONOUNSATURATED)
    10 WHOLE ALMONDS   1 TB. CHOPPED ALMONDS
    2 LARGE WHOLE PECANS ⅕ OZ. PECANS
    6 SM. WALNUTS   1 TB. CHOPPED WALNUTS
    6 SM. OTHER NUTS
    2 TB. FRESH SHREDDED COCONUT 1 TSP. DRIED, SHREDDED, UNSWEETENED COCONUT
  MEAT: (SATURATED)
    1 STRIP BACON   ¾″ CUBE SALT PORK
  SALAD DRESSINGS: (POLYUNSATURATED*)
    1 TSP. MAYONNAISE   2 TSP. MAYONNAISE-TYPE SALAD DRESSING
    1 TB. FRENCH DRESSING   2 TSP. ITALIAN DRESSING
    2 TSP. THOUSAND ISLAND DRESSING
    2 TB. LOW-CALORIE MAYONNAISE-TYPE SALAD DRESSING
    8 TB. LOW-CALORIE FRENCH DRESSING (1 FAT + 1 SUGAR)
    8 TB. LOW CALORIE ITALIAN DRESSING (1 FAT + ½ SUGAR)
    1 TB. IMITATION MAYONNAISE

*IF MADE FROM CORN, COTTONSEED, SAFFLOWER, SOYBEAN, OR SUNFLOWER OILS.

SUGAR EXCHANGES
ONE SUGAR EXCHANGE CONTAINS 12 GRAMS CARBOHYDRATE AND 48 CALORIES.
    1 TB. GRANULATED SUGAR   4 TSP. POWDERED SUGAR
    1 TB. BROWN SUGAR   ¼ OZ. HARD CANDY
    1 TB. LIGHT MOLASSES   4 OZ. SOFT DRINKS, CARBONATED
    1 TB. CORN OR MAPLE SYRUP   1 CUP SUGAR-COATED POPCORN
    1 TB. JAM OR JELLIES   ½ CUP LEMONADE
    2 TSP. HONEY   ⅙ CUP GELATIN DESSERT

ALCOHOL EXCHANGES

ONE ALCOHOL EXCHANGE CONTAINS 0–4 GRAMS CARBOHYDRATE, 4–5 GRAMS ALCOHOL, AND ABOUT 50 CALORIES.

4 FL. OZ. BEER	½ FL. OZ. WHISKEY OR RUM OR GIN OR VODKA
1 FL. OZ. DESSERT WINES	1½ FL. OZ. EGGNOG OR 2 FL. OZ. HIGHBALL
1½ FL. OZ. TABLE WINES	2 FL. OZ. GIN RICKEY ¼ MARTINI

SOURCE: "THE NUTRITIVE VALUE OF AMERICAN FOODS," AGRICULTURAL HANDBOOK NO. 456, WASHINGTON, D.C.: U.S. GPO, 1975.

TABLE 13 EXTRA-FUEL FOODS

FOOD	CAL	FAT EXCHANGES	FOOD	CAL	FAT EXCHANGES
ALCOHOLIC DRINKS			CRACKERS		
BEER, 12 OZ.	151	0	BUTTER, 1	17	0
GIN, RUM, VODKA, JIGGER	97	0	CHEESE, 1	15	0
WINE, DESSERT, 3½ OZ.	141	0	GRAHAM, 2	55	0
TABLE, 3½ OZ.	87	0	SALTINES, 1	12	0
SOFT DRINKS			SODA, 1	33	0
COLA TYPE, 12 OZ.	144	0	CREAM PUFFS, 3½" DIA.	303	3½
CREAM SODA, 12 OZ.	160	0	DOUGHNUTS		
FRUIT FLAVORED, 12 OZ.	171	0	CAKE TYPE, 3¼" DIA.	164	1½
GINGER ALE, 12 OZ.	113	0	YEAST, 3¼" DIA.	176	2
ROOT BEER, 12 OZ.	152	0	ECLAIRS, 1	239	2½
DIET DRINKS, 12 OZ.	0	0	GELATIN DESSERT, 1 CUP	315	0
CAKES			ICE CREAM, 1 CUP	257	2½
ANGEL FOOD, 2½" ARC	161	0	SOFT SERVE, 1 CUP	334	3½
BOSTON CREAM, 2½" ARC	208	1	ICE MILK, 1 CUP	199	1
CARAMEL W/ICING, 2½" ARC	398	3	SOFT SERVE, 1 CUP	266	1½
CHOCOLATE, ICING, 2½" ARC	365	3	JAMS, 1 TB.	54	0
FRUIT CAKE, ¼"×2"×½"	163	1	PIES (⅙)		
GINGERBREAD, 3"×3"×2"	371	2½	APPLE	404	3½
PLAIN, CHOC. ICING, 3"×3"×2"	453	3	BANANA CREAM	336	3
SPONGE, 2¼" ARC	131	½	CHERRY	412	3½
CANDY			CHOC. MERINGUE	383	3½
BUTTERSCOTCH, 1 OZ.	113	0	LEMON MERINGUE	357	3
CARAMELS, 1 OZ.	113	½	MINCE	428	3½
CHOCOLATE, SWEET, 1 OZ.	150	2	PUMPKIN	334	2½
CHOC. ALMONDS, 1 OZ.	161	2½	POPCORN, 1 CUP, POPPED	23	0
GUMDROPS, 1 OZ.	98	0	W/OIL, SALT	41	½
HARD, 1 OZ.	109	0	SUGAR COATED	134	½
JELLYBEANS (10), 1 OZ.	104	0	POTATO CHIPS, 10	114	1½
MARSHMALLOWS, 1 OZ.	90	0	PRETZELS, 8 OZ.	885	2
CHEWING GUM, 1 PC.	5	0	SUGAR, GRAN., 1 TB., 12 GRAMS	46	0
COOKIES			GRAN., 1 TSP., 4 GRAMS	15	0
ASSORTED, 1	42	0	SUGAR, POWD., 1 TB., 8 GRAMS	31	0
BROWNIES, 3"×1"×1"	97	1			
CHOC. CHIP, 1	50	½			
FIG BARS, 1	50	0			
GINGERSNAPS, 1, 2"	29	0			
MACAROONS, 1	90	1			
OATMEAL, 1	59	0			
SUGAR, 1	46	0			

TABLE 14   ENERGY EXPENDITURE

ACTIVITY	CAL/MIN.		
	125-LB. PERSON	150-LB. PERSON	175-LB. PERSON
BICYCLING, 5.5 MPH	4.2	5.1	5.9
RUNNING, 5.5 MPH	9.0	10.8	12.7
SWIMMING, 25 YD/MIN	5.0	6.1	7.1
WALKING, 2 MPH	2.9	3.5	4.2
4.5 MPH	5.5	6.7	7.8

TABLE 15   ACTIVITY EXPENDITURES
CALORIES PER MINUTE

ACTIVITY	BODY WEIGHTS				
	125 LB.	152 LB.	178 LB.	205 LB.	231 LB.
BADMINTON (RECREATIONAL)	5	6	7	8	9
BASEBALL (PLAYER)	4	5	6	6½	7
BICYCLING, 5.5 MPH (LEVEL)	4	5	6	7	8
BOWLING (NONSTOP)	6	7	8	9	10
CALISTHENICS	4	5	6	7	8
DANCE, MODERN (MODERATE)	3½	4	5	6	6½
DANCE, SQUARE	6	7	8	9	10
GOLF, TWOSOME	4	5	6	7	8
HIKING, 40-LB. PACK, 3 MPH	6	7	8	9	10½
HORSEBACK RIDING (TROT)	6	7	8	9	10
HORSESHOE PITCHING	3	3½	4	4½	5
MOUNTAIN CLIMBING	8	10	12	14	16
RACQUETBALL	8	10	12	13	15
POOL, BILLIARDS	1½	2	2	2½	3
RUNNING, 11 MIN. MILE, 5.5 MPH	9	11	13	15	17
RUNNING, STATIONARY, 140 STEPS PER MINUTE	20	25	29	33	38
SKIING, LEVEL, 5 MPH	10	12	14	16	18
SWIMMING, 25 YD./MIN.	5	6	7	8	9
TABLE TENNIS	3	4	4½	5	6
TENNIS (RECREATIONAL)	6	7	8	9	10
WALKING, 2 MPH	3	3½	4	4½	5
WALKING, 4.5 MPH	5½	7	8	9	10

ADAPTED FROM: "Calorie Expenditure Per Minute for Selected Exercises," in *Fitness for Life, an Individualized Approach,* by Allsen, Harrison, and Vance, Dubuque, Iowa: William C. Brown, 1976, p. 89.

(AGES 25 AND OVER)*

HEIGHT (WITH SHOES, 2-INCH HEELS)		WEIGHT IN POUNDS ACCORDING TO FRAME (IN INDOOR CLOTHING)		
		SMALL FRAME	MEDIUM FRAME	LARGE FRAME
FEET	INCHES			
4	10	92– 98	96–107	104–119
4	11	94–101	98–110	106–122
5	0	96–104	101–113	109–125
5	1	99–107	104–116	112–128
5	2	102–110	107–119	115–131
5	3	105–113	110–122	118–134
5	4	108–116	113–126	121–138
5	5	111–119	116–130	125–142
5	6	114–123	120–135	129–146
5	7	118–127	124–139	133–150
5	8	122–131	128–143	137–154
5	9	126–135	132–147	141–158
5	10	130–140	136–151	145–163
5	11	134–144	140–155	149–168
6	0	138–148	144–159	153–173

NOTE: For girls between 18 and 25, subtract 1 pound for each year under 25. Courtesy of the Metropolitan Life Insurance Company, New York, N.Y. Derived from data of the 1959 Build and Blood Pressure Study, Society of Actuaries.

DESIRABLE WEIGHTS FOR MEN
(AGES 25 AND OVER)*

HEIGHT (WITH SHOES, 2-INCH HEELS)		WEIGHT IN POUNDS ACCORDING TO FRAME (IN INDOOR CLOTHING)		
		SMALL FRAME	MEDIUM FRAME	LARGE FRAME
FEET	INCHES			
5	2	112–120	118–129	126–141
5	3	115–123	121–133	129–144
5	4	118–126	124–136	132–148
5	5	121–129	127–139	135–152
5	6	124–133	130–143	138–156
5	7	128–137	134–147	142–161
5	8	132–141	138–152	147–166
5	9	136–145	142–156	151–170
5	10	140–150	146–160	155–174
5	11	144–154	150–165	159–179
6	0	148–158	154–170	164–184
6	1	152–162	158–175	168–189
6	2	156–167	162–180	173–194
6	3	160–171	167–185	178–199
6	4	164–175	172–190	182–204

*Courtesy of the Metropolitan Life Insurance Company, New York, N.Y. Derived from data of the 1959 Build and Blood Pressure Study, Society of Actuaries.

Determining Recommended Body Weight

A method of estimating recommended body weight from body measurements is given below: To make the measurements, it is first necessary to construct a sliding caliper. For this you need a yardstick at a 90-degree angle. Make a groove the width of the yardstick in the other board, so that the board can slide along the yardstick. See Figure 14.

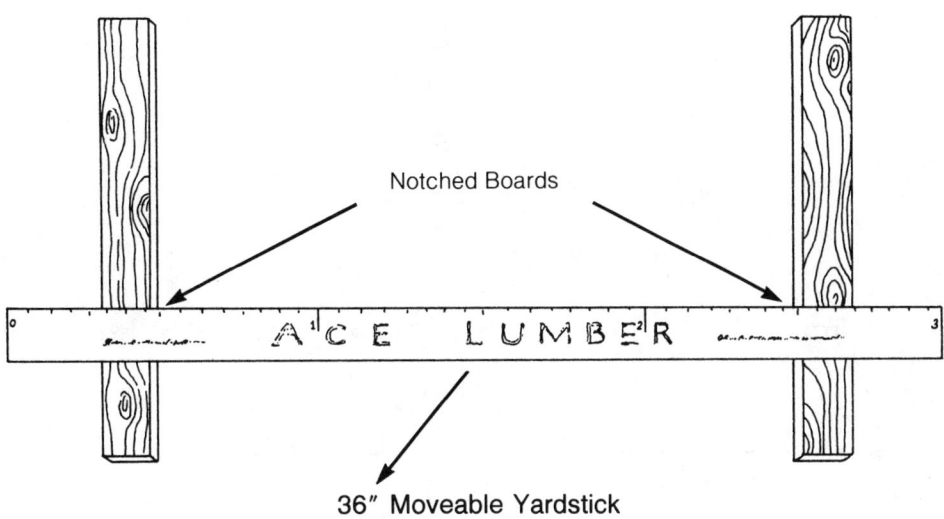

Notched Boards

ACE LUMBER

36″ Moveable Yardstick

Fig. 14

To calculate your recommended body weight, three measurements are needed. The first is an accurate measurement of your height. Stand with your heels next to a flat wall. Have a helper place a ruler flat on your head and mark the wall where the ruler touches. Measure the distance from the floor to the mark; record the inches.

The second measurement is your shoulder width: Have a helper stand behind you and place the stationary side of the caliper on the left edge of the shoulder bone (not the arm bone), and then slide the moveable side of the caliper to the right edge of the shoulder bone. See Figure 15A. Record the distance in inches.

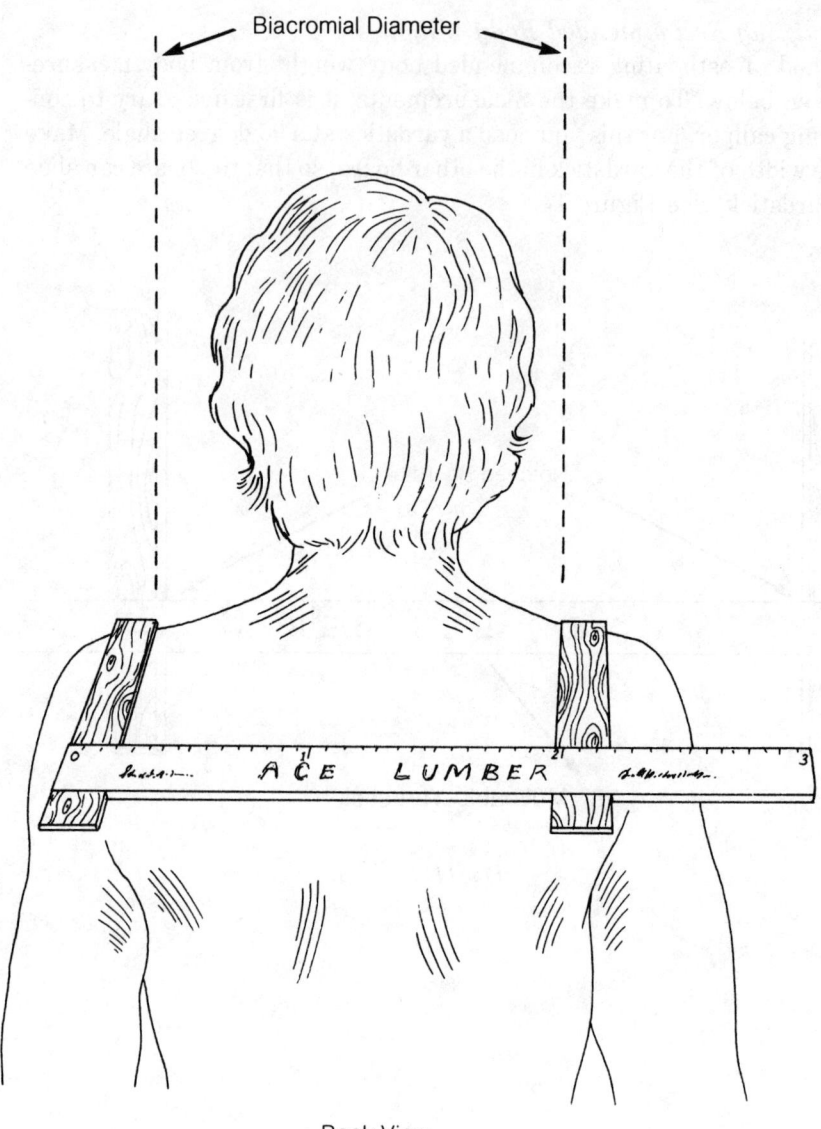

Back View

Fig. 15A

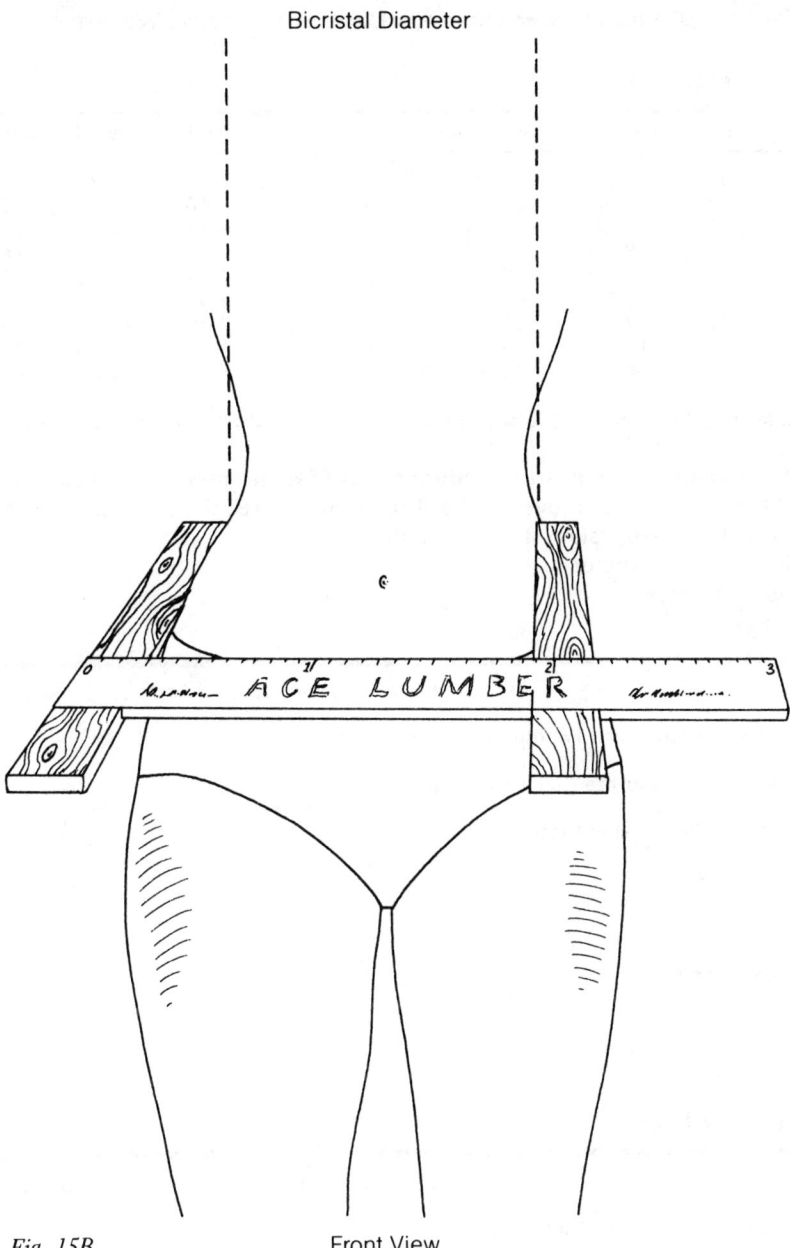

Bicristal Diameter

Fig. 15B

Front View

The third measurement is the width of your hip bone. Have a helper stand in front of you and place the stationary side of the caliper on the right edge of your hip bone. (Press hard, trying to have the board touch the bone as closely as possible.) Then place the sliding side of the caliper on the left edge of your hip bone. See Figure 15B. Record the measurement in inches.

TABLE 17 CONVERSION FACTORS FOR CALCULATING IDEAL WEIGHT

		MALES					FEMALES		
AGE	HGHT.	S.W.C.F.[1]	H.W.C.F.[2]	CONSTANT	AGE	HGHT.	S.W.C.F.[1]	H.W.C.F.[2]	CONSTANT
3– 4	1.56	2.07	.78	48.69	3– 4	1.45	1.01	1.34	40.59
5– 6	1.62	2.51	1.90	66.11	5– 6	1.68	2.40	.84	59.84
7– 8	2.85	2.57	.34	114.14	7– 8	2.07	4.14	4.75	126.30
9–10	2.51	6.48	3.19	166.36	9–10	2.79	4.64	2.07	147.75
11–12	2.46	7.43	5.20	193.12	11–12	3.19	4.81	6.59	191.29
13–14	3.02	8.33	5.36	246.09	13–14	.89	12.68	6.59	182.84
15–16	.67	8.27	17.77	217.21	15–16	.84	7.66	15.74	199.14
17–19	2.63	10.34	11.23	314.73	17–19	1.45	9.28	10.84	207.68
20+	1.84	7.10	6.09	145.07	20+	1.12	8.94	9.28	168.01

NOTE: Since skeletal growth is completed before age 30, the 20+ age group can be used for all ages above 20.

Conversion factors adapted from: **An Introduction to Measurement in Physical Education,** Vol. II, edited by H. J. Montoye, p. 53. Copyright © 1970 by Phi Epsilon Kappa Fraternity. Reprinted by permission of the publisher.

[1]shoulder-width conversion factor

[2]hip-width conversion factor

RECORD FORM

NAME_____ SEX_____ AGE_____ DATE_____

1. HEIGHT _____ × HEIGHT CONVERSION FACTOR _____ = _____

2. SHOULDER WIDTH _____ × SHOULDER CONVERSION FACTOR _____ = _____

3. HIP WIDTH _____ × HIP CONVERSION FACTOR _____ = _____

4. SUBTOTAL: ITEMS 1, 2, 3 = _____

5. CONSTANT = _____

6. ESTIMATED RECOMMENDED WEIGHT. SUBTRACT ITEM 5 FROM ITEM 4 = _____

SAMPLE RECORD FORM

NAME_____ SEX_____ AGE_____ DATE_____

1. HEIGHT _____ × HEIGHT CONVERSION FACTOR _____ = _____

2. SHOULDER WIDTH _____ × SHOULDER CONVERSION FACTOR _____ = _____

3. HIP WIDTH _____ × HIP CONVERSION FACTOR _____ = _____

4. SUBTOTAL: ITEMS 1, 2, 3 = _____

5. CONSTANT = _____

6. ESTIMATED RECOMMENDED WEIGHT. SUBTRACT ITEM 5 FROM ITEM 4 = _____

ADAPTED FROM: *Fitness for Life, an Individual Approach,* by Allsen, Harrison, and Vance, William C. Brown Co., Dubuque, Iowa: 1976, p. 13.

APPENDIX C.

Blank Record Forms

WORKSHEET #1. SUPPORT AND REWARDS

WEIGHT-CONTROL CLASS AT _____

      STARTING DATE_____TIME_____

OR/AND

      FRIENDS—THE PERSONS IN THIS GROUP WILL BE:

NAME	ADDRESS

REWARDS—THINGS I LIKE TO DO:

_____

_____

_____

_____

_____

_____

174

REWARDS—THINGS I WOULD LIKE TO HAVE (NONFOOD):

_____

_____

_____

_____

_____

WORKSHEET #2. FOOD AND BEHAVIOR RECORD

NAME _____ DATES _____

DATE TIMES	PLACE	PHYSICAL POSITION	WITH WHOM?	ASSOC. ACTIVITY	MOOD	HUNGER	FOOD AND AMOUNT

IDEAL WEIGHT
WEIGHT RESPONSE

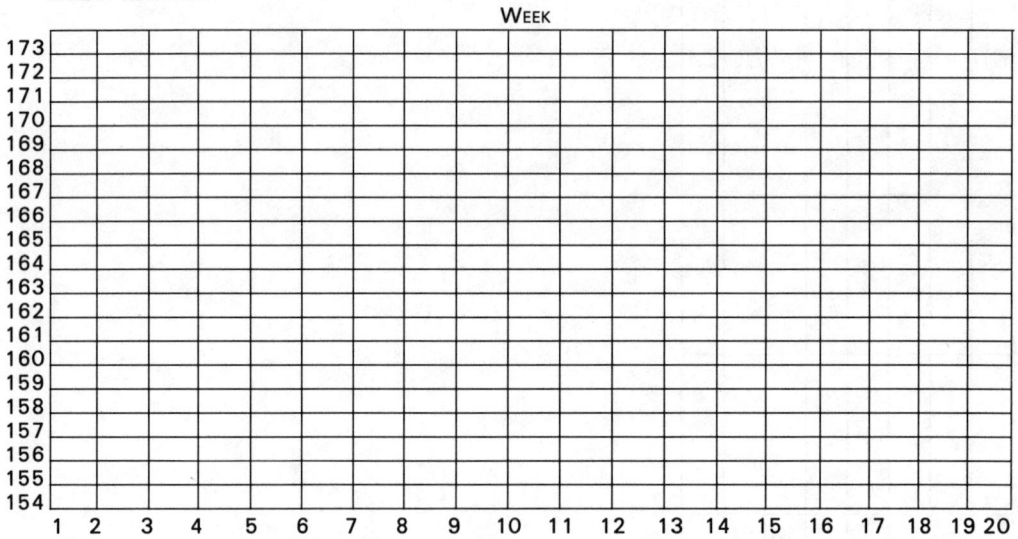

MEASUREMENT RESPONSE

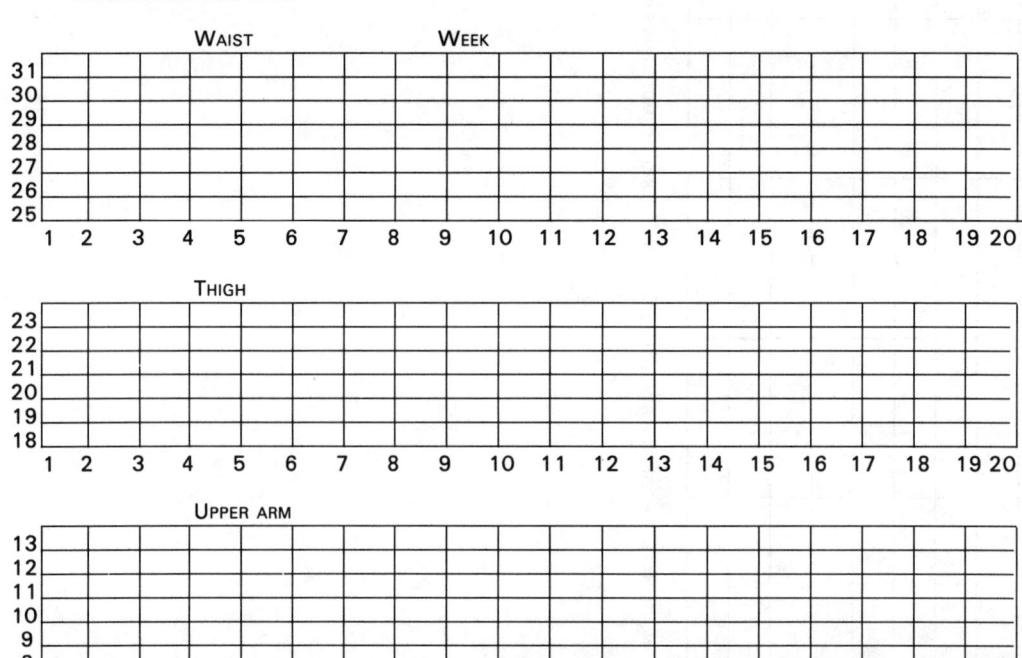

WORKSHEET #4. WALKING RECORD

WEEK 1. DATES_____

DAY	TIME STARTED	TIME ENDED	WITH WHOM	WHERE

WEEK 2. DATES_____

DAY	TIME STARTED	TIME ENDED	WITH WHOM	WHERE

WEEK 3. DATES_____

DAY	TIME STARTED	TIME ENDED	WITH WHOM	WHERE

WEEK 4. DATES_____

REWARD SELECTED_____

REWARDS EARNED AND OBTAINED WHEN_____

_____

180

WORKSHEET #5. MEAL-PLANNING RECORD   NAME____

DAY	BREAKFAST	LUNCH	DINNER	TOTAL EXCHANGES
SUNDAY	1 MILK, 1 MEAT, 1 FAT 1 BREAD, 1 FRUIT	1 MILK, 1 MEAT, 1 FAT 1 BREAD, 2 FRUIT, 1 VEG.	0 MILK, 3 MEAT, 1 FAT 1 BREAD, 1 FRUIT, 2 VEG.	2 MILK, 5 MEAT, 3 FAT 3 BREAD, 4 FRUIT, 3 VEG.
MONDAY				MILK___ MEAT___ FAT___ BREAD___ FRUIT___ VEG.___
TUESDAY				MILK___ MEAT___ FAT___ BREAD___ FRUIT___ VEG.___
				MILK___ MEAT___ FAT___ BREAD___ FRUIT___ VEG.___

WEDNESDAY

MILK___
MEAT___
FAT___
BREAD___
FRUIT___
VEG.___

THURSDAY

MILK___
MEAT___
FAT___
BREAD___
FRUIT___
VEG.___

FRIDAY

MILK___
MEAT___
FAT___
BREAD___
FRUIT___
VEG.___

SATURDAY

MILK___
MEAT___
FAT___
BREAD___
FRUIT___
VEG.___

DATE	ACTIVITY	TIME STARTED	TIME ENDED	TEN-SECOND PULSE RATE

WORKSHEET #7.   TONING EXERCISE RECORD   NAME_____

DATE	EXERCISE	MINS.	DATE	EXERCISE	MINS.

REWARDS: STATE DATE AND TYPE OF REWARD

NAME_____   WEEK OF_____

DATE TIME	PLACE	FOOD AND AMOUNT	CALORIES	ENERGY EQUIVALENT	E. F. PRICE PAID TIME

WORKSHEET #9. ANALYSIS OF FOOD-AND-BEHAVIOR RECORD

HOW MANY TIMES EACH DAY DID YOU:	SUN		MON		TUE		WED		THU		FRI		SAT		TOTAL	
	WEEK 1	WEEK 2	WEEK 1	WEEK 2	WEEK 1	WEEK 2	WEEK 1	WEEK 2	WEEK 1	WEEK 2	WEEK 1	WEEK 2	WEEK 1	WEEK 2	WEEK 1	WEEK 2
1. EAT SOMETHING?																
2. EAT EMPTY-CALORIE FOODS?																
3. EAT NOT SITTING AT A TABLE?																
4. EAT WHILE DOING OTHER THINGS?																
5. EAT ALONE AT NONMEALTIMES?																
6. EAT WITH A FRIEND AT NONMEALTIMES?																
7. EAT WHEN YOU WERE FEELING BORED?																
8. EAT WHEN FEELING RESTLESS?																
9. EAT WHEN FEELING ANGRY OR UNHAPPY?																
10. EAT WHEN FEELING WORRIED?																
11. EAT WHEN FEELING LONELY?																
12. GORGE YOURSELF WITH ONE CERTAIN FOOD?																
13. EAT LARGE AMOUNTS OF FOOD?																
14. EAT WHEN YOU WERE NOT HUNGRY?																

GOAL-SETTING CHART

MY GOALS WILL BE:

1.

2.

3.

I WILL REARRANGE MY ENVIRONMENT BY:

1.

2.

3.

I WILL PRACTICE:

1.

2.

3.

4.

5.

I WILL REWARD MYSELF FOR SUCCESS BY:

M	T	W	T	F	S	S

1.

2.

3.

I WILL EXTEND MY GOAL:

	M	T	W	T	F	S	S		M	T	W	T	F	S	S
1.															
2.															
3.															
4.															
5.															

WORKSHEET #12. CONTROLLING MOODS WITH SUBSTITUTE ACTIVITIES

SUBSTITUTE ACTIVITIES:
PLEASANT ACTIVITIES

_____

_____

_____

_____

_____

NECESSARY ACTIVITIES:

_____

_____

_____

_____

_____

188

SITUATIONS WHERE ACTIVITY WILL BE USED:

1. _____

2. _____

3. _____

4. _____

5. _____

6. _____

7. _____

8. _____

9. _____

10. _____

11. _____

12. _____

13. _____

14. _____

15. _____

SITUATIONS WHEN ACTIVITY WAS ACTUALLY USED:

1. _____

2. _____

3. _____

4. _____

5. _____

6. _____

7. _____

8. _____

9. _____

10. _____

GOALS:

1. _____

_____

2. _____

_____

3. _____

_____

SPECIFIC PLANS:

_____

_____

_____

_____

_____

_____

_____

WORKSHEET #14. MY OWN ACTIVITY RECORD   NAME_____

DATE	ACTIVITY	TIME STARTED	TIME ENDED	TEN-SECOND PULSE RATE

DATE	ACTIVITY	TIME STARTED	TIME ENDED	TEN-SECOND PULSE RATE

WORKSHEET #14. MY OWN ACTIVITY RECORD   NAME_____

DATE	ACTIVITY	TIME STARTED	TIME ENDED	TEN-SECOND PULSE RATE

DATE	ACTIVITY	TIME STARTED	TIME ENDED	TEN-SECOND PULSE RATE

WORKSHEET #14. MY OWN ACTIVITY RECORD   NAME_____

DATE	ACTIVITY	TIME STARTED	TIME ENDED	TEN-SECOND PULSE RATE

WORKSHEET #15. MAINTENANCE MEAL-PLANNING RECORD

NAME _____

DAY	BREAKFAST	LUNCH	DINNER	TOTAL EXCHANGES
	1 MILK, 1 MEAT, 1 FAT 1 BREAD, 1 FRUIT	1 MILK, 1 MEAT, 1 FAT 1 BREAD, 2 FRUIT, 1 VEG.	0 MILK, 3 MEAT, 1 FAT 1 BREAD, 1 FRUIT, 2 VEG.	2 MILK, 5 MEAT, 3 FAT 3 BREAD, 4 FRUIT, 3 VEG.
SUNDAY				MILK__ MEAT__ FAT__ BREAD__ FRUIT__ VEG.__
MONDAY				MILK__ MEAT__ FAT__ BREAD__ FRUIT__ VEG.__
TUESDAY				MILK__ MEAT__ FAT__ BREAD__ FRUIT__ VEG.__

WEDNESDAY

MILK___
MEAT___
FAT___
BREAD___
FRUIT___
VEG.___

THURSDAY

MILK___
MEAT___
FAT___
BREAD___
FRUIT___
VEG.___

FRIDAY

MILK___
MEAT___
FAT___
BREAD___
FRUIT___
VEG.___

SATURDAY

MILK___
MEAT___
FAT___
BREAD___
FRUIT___
VEG.___

WORKSHEET #15. MAINTENANCE MEAL-PLANNING RECORD

NAME _____

DAY	BREAKFAST	LUNCH	DINNER	TOTAL EXCHANGES
SUNDAY	1 MILK, 1 MEAT, 1 FAT 1 BREAD, 1 FRUIT	1 MILK, 1 MEAT, 1 FAT 1 BREAD, 2 FRUIT, 1 VEG.	0 MILK, 3 MEAT, 1 FAT 1 BREAD, 1 FRUIT, 2 VEG.	2 MILK, 5 MEAT, 3 FAT 3 BREAD, 4 FRUIT, 3 VEG. MILK__ MEAT__ FAT__ BREAD__ FRUIT__ VEG.__
MONDAY				MILK__ MEAT__ FAT__ BREAD__ FRUIT__ VEG.__
TUESDAY				MILK__ MEAT__ FAT__ BREAD__ FRUIT__ VEG.__

WEDNESDAY

MILK___
MEAT___
FAT___
BREAD___
FRUIT___
VEG.___

THURSDAY

MILK___
MEAT___
FAT___
BREAD___
FRUIT___
VEG.___

FRIDAY

MILK___
MEAT___
FAT___
BREAD___
FRUIT___
VEG.___

SATURDAY

MILK___
MEAT___
FAT___
BREAD___
FRUIT___
VEG.___

201

WORKSHEET #15. MAINTENANCE MEAL-PLANNING RECORD

NAME_____

DAY	BREAKFAST	LUNCH	DINNER	TOTAL EXCHANGES
	1 MILK, 1 MEAT, 1 FAT 1 BREAD, 1 FRUIT	1 MILK, 1 MEAT, 1 FAT 1 BREAD, 2 FRUIT, 1 VEG.	0 MILK, 3 MEAT, 1 FAT 1 BREAD, 1 FRUIT, 2 VEG.	2 MILK, 5 MEAT, 3 FAT 3 BREAD, 4 FRUIT, 3 VEG.
SUNDAY				MILK___ MEAT___ FAT___ BREAD___ FRUIT___ VEG.___
MONDAY				MILK___ MEAT___ FAT___ BREAD___ FRUIT___ VEG.___
TUESDAY				MILK___ MEAT___ FAT___ BREAD___ FRUIT___ VEG.___

WEDNESDAY

MILK___
MEAT___
FAT___
BREAD___
FRUIT___
VEG.___

THURSDAY

MILK___
MEAT___
FAT___
BREAD___
FRUIT___
VEG.___

FRIDAY

MILK___
MEAT___
FAT___
BREAD___
FRUIT___
VEG.___

SATURDAY

MILK___
MEAT___
FAT___
BREAD___
FRUIT___
VEG.___

WORKSHEET #15. Maintenance Meal-Planning Record   NAME____

DAY	BREAKFAST	LUNCH	DINNER	TOTAL EXCHANGES
SUNDAY	1 MILK, 1 MEAT, 1 FAT 1 BREAD, 1 FRUIT	1 MILK, 1 MEAT, 1 FAT 1 BREAD, 2 FRUIT, 1 VEG.	0 MILK, 3 MEAT, 1 FAT 1 BREAD, 1 FRUIT, 2 VEG.	2 MILK, 5 MEAT, 3 FAT 3 BREAD, 4 FRUIT, 3 VEG.
MONDAY				MILK__ MEAT__ FAT__ BREAD__ FRUIT__ VEG.__
TUESDAY				MILK__ MEAT__ FAT__ BREAD__ FRUIT__ VEG.__

WEDNESDAY

MILK___
MEAT___
FAT___
BREAD___
FRUIT___
VEG.___

THURSDAY

MILK___
MEAT___
FAT___
BREAD___
FRUIT___
VEG.___

FRIDAY

MILK___
MEAT___
FAT___
BREAD___
FRUIT___
VEG.___

SATURDAY

MILK___
MEAT___
FAT___
BREAD___
FRUIT___
VEG.___

Index

Food and behavior, 69, 72–73, 110–18
  analysis of worksheet on, 110–11
  external stimuli, 112–13
  goal-setting chart, 114–15
  mood-eating problems, 115–18
  record keeping, 72–73
  worksheet, 72–73
  See also Behavior modification
Food and Behavior Record (worksheet),
  72–73
  analysis of, 110–11
Food and Nutrition Board, 12
Food conversion, 24–32
  cells and, 27–28
  cellular conversion, 29–32
  digestion, 24–25
  enzymes and cofactors, 28–29
  nutrients, absorption of, 26–27
Food exchanges, 79–83, 98–99
  alcohol, 83
  bread-cereal-starchy-vegetable, 81–82
  explained, 79–80
  fat, 81
  fruit, 82
  meat, 80
  milk, 80
  nonnutrients, 83
  recipes and, 98–99
  sugar, 82
  table, 84–85
  vegetables, 82
Food labels, 12
Food preparation and preservation, 83–
  86
  cooking at low temperatures, 86
  fat on meat, 86
  fruit, 86
  salt, 86
  sugar, 86
Food presence stimuli, 44–45
  Principle/Procedure (table), 45
Food utilization, 5, 7–8
Fruit exchanges, 82

Glycogen, 31
Goal-Setting Chart (worksheet), 114–15
Goiter, 17
Gout, 19

Heart disease, 21
Heart rate, 101–2
High-fat diets, 53
High-fiber diets, 53
High-protein diets, 52–53

Hormones, 7–8
  insulin, 8
  thyroxine, 8
Human chorionic gonadotropin (HCG), 56
Hypertension, 18
Hypothalamus, 5–6
  appestat, 6
  "feeding center," 6
  "satiety center," 6

Ideal weight, 74, 131
Inactivity, 8–9
Insulin, 8
Iron, 17
Iron deficiency anemia, 17

Ketosis, 19

Lactation. *See* Pregnancy
Lactic acid, 31
Last Chance Diet, The, 51
Laxatives, 55
Lifelong Activity Program, 119–21
  duration, 120
  frequency, 120
  inclement weather and, 121
  intensity, 120
  type of activity, 120
  worksheet, 122–23
Lipoproteins, 21
Liquid-protein diet, 52
Loneliness, 47
Low-carbohydrate diets, 52

Maintenance diets, 121–25
  daily calorie determination, 121
  examples (tables), 123–24
  weighing in, 124
Maintenance Exchange Diets (table),
  123–24
Meal planning, 87–99
  cafeterias, 98
  dining with friends, 98
  extra fuel foods, 87
  fast-food restaurants, 98
  "going off" the plan, 91
  1000-calorie exchange diet, 87
  1500-calorie exchange diet, 87
  recipes and exchanges, 98–99
  reduced calorie diets, 87–89
  restaurants, 91
  salt, 89
  snack bars, 98
  sweeteners, 87–89

Refined sugar, 70
Restaurants, 91
Restlessness, 46

Saccharin, 146–47
Salt, 17–18, 86, 89
  in food preparation, 86
"Satiety center," 6
Saturated fats, 21
Scurvy, 15
70 percent training rate, 101–2
Signals for eating, 7
Snack bars, 98
Sodium. *See* Salt
Sugar
  in food preparation, 86
  refined, 20
Sugar exchanges, 82
Sulfur, 15
Support and Rewards (worksheet), 70–71
Surgery. *See* Bypass surgery

Teen-agers. *See* Adolescence
Thyroid extracts, 56
Thyroxine, 8
Toning Exercise Record (worksheet),
  108
Toning exercises, 104–6
  deep knee-bends, 104
  leg-overs, 106
  push-off wall, 105
  standing twists, 105
  worksheet, 108
Trace minerals, 15, 18

Vegetable exchanges, 82
Vegetarian diets, 53
Vitamin B, 15
Vitamin C, 15, 144
Vitamin D, 15, 144
Vitamin E, 15
Vitamin K, 15, 144
Vitamins, 13–15, 87, 144
  deficiencies, 13, 15
  disease and, 15
  excess intake, 15
  fat soluble, 13, 15
  supplements, 87
  table, 14
  toxic effects, 15
  water soluble, 13, 15

Walking program, 60, 76–78, 104
  physical benefits, 76
  psychological benefits, 76
  regularity in following, 76
  worksheet, 77–78
Walking Program Record (worksheet),
  77–78
Water, 13
Weight-loss program. *See* Bio-plan for
  weight control
Weight and Measurement Record (worksheet), 75
Worry, 47

Yang-Van Itallie diet study, 54–55

Zinc, 17